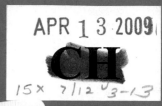

# FITNESS
## MADE SIMPLE

# FITNESS MADE SIMPLE

## THE POWER TO CHANGE YOUR BODY
## THE POWER TO CHANGE YOUR LIFE

# JOHN BASEDOW

### WITH TOM McGRATH

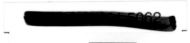

New York   Chicago   San Francisco   Lisbon   London   Madrid   Mexico City
Milan   New Delhi   San Juan   Seoul   Singapore   Sydney   Toronto

**Library of Congress Cataloging-in-Publication Data**

Basedow, John.
    Fitness made simple / John Basedow with Tom McGrath.
       p.   cm.
    ISBN-13: 978-0-07-149708-4 (alk. paper)
     1. Physical fitness.   2. Exercise.   3. Muscle strength.   4. Nutrition.
  I. McGrath, Tom.   II. Title.
  GV481.B275   2007
  613.7—dc22

                          2007025678

1  2  3  4  5  6  7  8  9  10  11  12  13  14  15  16  17  18  19  20   DOC/DOC   0  9  8  7

ISBN  978-0-07-149708-4 (book and DVD)
MHID     0-07-149708-0 (book and DVD)
ISBN  978-0-07-154461-0 (book alone)
MHID     0-07-154461-5 (book alone)

Interior design by Think Design Group LLC
Photographs on pages 126–130, 132–133, 136–137, 139, 141, 145, 148–173, 175–186, 190–216, 220–230 by Mitch Mandel
Photographs on pages 124–125, 131, 134–135, 138, 140, 142, 146–147, 187–189, 218–219 by Yolanda Perez

McGraw-Hill books are available at special quantity discounts to use as premiums and sales promotions, or for use in corporate training programs. For more information, please write to the Director of Special Sales, Professional Publishing, McGraw-Hill, Two Penn Plaza, New York, NY 10121-2298. Or contact your local bookstore.

This book is for educational purposes. It is not intended as a substitute for individual fitness, health, and medical advice. Please consult a qualified health care professional for individual health and medical advice. Neither McGraw-Hill nor the author shall have any responsibility for any adverse effects that arise directly or indirectly as a result of the information provided in this book.

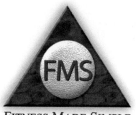

**FITNESS MADE SIMPLE**

This book is dedicated to my mom, along with
all of the FMS members and fans, who inspire me
beyond belief. Thanks to your support,
I'm living my dream and I feel incredibly blessed that
the FMS programs are helping thousands of other
men and women achieve their dreams as well.
Always remember, as long as you believe in yourself,
you can accomplish anything.

# CONTENTS

**PART 1**

## Take Control of Your Body

**PART 2**

## The Fitness Triangle

**PART 3**

## Change Your Body, Change Your Life

# PREFACE

My name is John Basedow or, as I'm referred to everywhere from national television to the *New York Times*, "Fitness Celebrity John Basedow." When I started Fitness Made Simple, I realized that it was a way for me to achieve two big goals. First, it allowed me to tell the world how fitness changes lives in incredibly powerful ways. Fitness transformed my life just as it can transform yours. Second, Fitness Made Simple gave me the opportunity to touch people through television, something I've wanted to do for as long as I can remember.

I've been lucky enough to reach thousands of people over the past few years with my numerous bestselling workout and nutrition videos, from *Fitness Made Simple: Unlock Your Potential* to *Six Pack Abs*. However, until now I haven't been able to put together in one place *everything* I know about the power of following a fitness lifestyle. That's why I wrote this book—to tell the full story of how fitness dramatically improved my life and to lay out in detail how it can do the same for you.

If you're new to Fitness Made Simple, you'll find everything you need here, from my basic philosophy about fitness to complete nutrition and exercise plans that will help you change your body. If you're already famil-iar with Fitness Made Simple through some of our videos, you'll find lots of brand-new information and advice I've never shared before, from a detailed meal plan and expanded exercise program to more than 20 FMS Success Stories. They're the ultimate proof that proper diet and exercise can pro-foundly improve not only the way you look but, even more important, the way you feel about yourself.

Whether you're a teenager, a grandparent, or somewhere in between, Fitness Made Simple is all about giving you power—the power to change your body, the power to change your life, the power to be better. That power is now in your hands.

# ACKNOWLEDGMENTS

Many thanks to . . .

- Linda Basedow, the best mom a son could have, for always keeping promises and teaching me how to do the same.
- Carline Mordan, my rock, for believing in me even when I didn't. You make every day special just by being in it. You are magic, period.
- Pat Riches, Fran Capo, Virginia Greenfield, and Justin Zickmund (aka the Angel Crew), along with all of the gang at Fitness Made Simple and "John Basedow TV," for being such great friends who have helped to turn my dreams into reality. You challenge me to think outside the box and, more important, give me the comfort of knowing I'm not alone because I have your support in everything I do.
- Paquita McCray, for sharing some of the best times of my life and inspiring me to never quit.
- Mummie, Poppie, and the whole Jean-Charles clan, for being such amazing people and making me part of the family. I love you all so much.
- All of the many people who ever doubted me, told me *no*, and tried to impose their limitations on my abilities. You made me stronger and showed me that the power to accomplish anything was always within me. Now that realization is a gift I can share with others.
- Jeremy Katz, for being the best agent and friend I could ever hope for. You are truly an amazing person, and I can't thank you enough for getting me involved in this crazy world of book publishing.
- Tom McGrath, for being such a great guy and the most talented cowriter I've ever worked with.
- Johanna Bowman, my editor, and all of my new friends at McGraw-Hill, for believing in me and my vision. You helped make this book possible and turned writing it into one of the most rewarding experiences of my life.

# TAKE CONTROL OF YOUR BODY

———

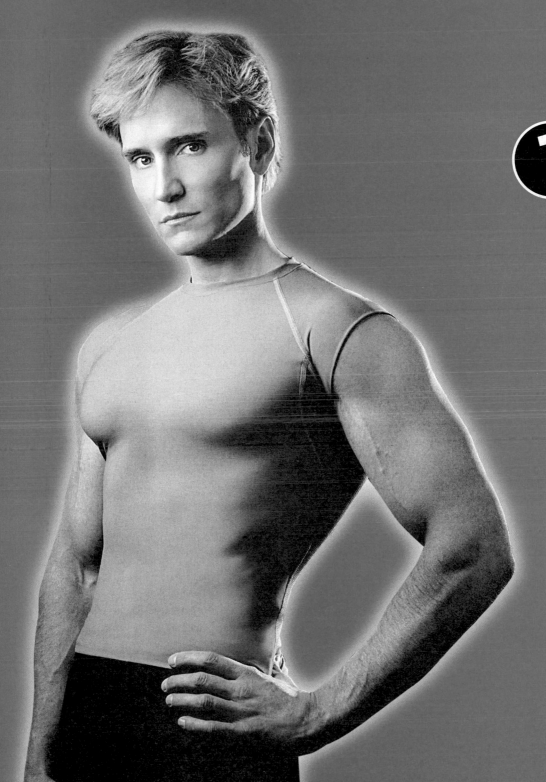

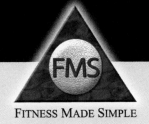

**FITNESS MADE SIMPLE**

# THE POWER TO CHANGE YOUR LIFE

Today's failure has no bearing on tomorrow's success.

Ever heard that before? If you've seen any of the thousands of Fitness Made Simple commercials I've put on TV over the past few years or watched any of the bestselling videos I've made, I'm betting you have. It's a mantra I repeat over and over. It sums up what Fitness Made Simple is all about: *what you are today doesn't necessarily indicate what you'll be tomorrow.* It's an idea that's helped thousands of people of all ages, shapes, and sizes change not only their bodies but also their lives.

And now it's going to help you.

By the way, that particular saying—a "John-ism," the media calls it, and you'll see many of them sprinkled throughout this book—isn't something I say just because it sounds good or because I read it in some dusty old tome on philosophy. No, I say it because I believe it, and I believe it because I've lived it. I know what it is to be at your lowest point and to lift yourself out of that quagmire.

Let me take you back a few years, when my life could only be described as a barrelful of zeroes. I was a couple of years out of school and living off the puny residuals of a TV show I'd been part of when I was in college. Well, I guess you can call it living. I didn't have a job, didn't have many prospects, and was more than $60,000 in debt. Things were so bad that when the bill collectors called—and let me tell you, they called a lot—I'd pretend I was somebody else. "Mr. Basedow not here," I'd respond in my best fake foreign accent. "I just clean. You call back some other time." Then I'd change my phone number. Of course, you can't dodge bill collectors forever. I finally took out a loan to pay my mortgage. How pathetic is that? It's like using Visa to pay MasterCard.

Things weren't always so bad for me. For most of my life I was a driven, goal-oriented individual. As a teenager I played tennis on the junior circuit. In high school I studied hard and became salutatorian of my class. In college a partner and I started a television magazine show called "Images." We did quite well, syndicating it out of my parents' basement and getting it aired on more than 200 stations in the United States, along with countless others in more than 30 countries. It was a great three years, and the show succeeded beyond my wildest expectations. I made a lot of connections in the TV industry and even met Oprah, Regis, and a lot of other big-time TV hosts.

But then, like most shows, "Images" ran out of steam, and my life seemed to run out of steam with it. Oh, I still had plenty of energy, but I didn't have a road map for where I was going.

And the body that had once made me a pretty good tennis player? It had become soft and chubby. I looked like a bowling pin on legs. It wasn't

# JOHN-ISM

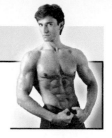

There is nothing good about being normal. Normal is average, and who the hell wants to be average?

hard to figure out why. Every night after midnight I'd go directly from my office to the White Castle drive-through, where I'd buy a sack of 10 White Castle burgers—Belly Bombers, in the argot of the time. Given my financial state it wasn't always easy to pay for them. More than once I crawled around on the floor of my car, looking for loose change to pay the bill. But once I found it—well, you couldn't have seen a bigger smile on my face. I never failed to finish the whole bag before I got home, and it was only a 15-minute drive! Not that the burgers totally satisfied me. I'd usually devour three-quarters of an Entenmann's chocolate brownie cake and a big jug of milk before I went to bed.

No wonder I couldn't see my abs.

After more than a few miles on that supersized highway, I eventually decided to try and get myself into shape, but that only made things worse. Over the course of a year, I tried every diet known to man: high-carb, low-fat, vegetarian, grapefruit. I jogged, cycled, pounded stair steppers and heavy weights. I tried Olympic lifting, Nautilus, circuit training, free weights, balls, and bands. And you know what? I looked lousy. The lifting increased my muscle mass a little, but the disaster that was my eating plan hid it all under a thick layer of fat. I was as smooth as a bar of soap.

All in all it was a pretty lethal combination: no career success and failure at the one personal goal I had set for myself—getting a better body. I hated to be around people because I felt like such a loser. I stayed away from family and friends because I didn't want to hear their questions about what I was up to or, worse, be on the receiving end of their pity.

# JOHN-ISM

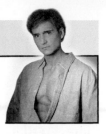

Every successful person has failed in the past. They just never let those failures stand in their way.

The low point for me came at Christmastime that year. I had a big tree I bought on sale the previous year. On Christmas day my family was all together for our celebration. For one day I figured I could handle being around them. Then my aunt called for her yearly chat with us all. As she spoke to all the members of the family, I heard them recount their successes as she asked about the high points of the year. Finally, it was my turn. I held the phone up to my ear.

"John."

Pause.

"I hear you've got a really big tree."

That was it, my big success for the year. For the first time I felt as bad as I looked. Sometimes it takes an outside perspective—like my aunt's—to really shine a light on how far I was from where I wanted to be.

But that was the day I made a vow to myself: *today's failures have no bearing on tomorrow's success.*

FITNESS MADE SIMPLE

Looking back I realize that was a point where I could have given up. A lot of people do. They say, "It ain't gonna get any better. I guess this is what I'm stuck with. I'll make the best of it." They come down with a disease I call *settle-itis*. They settle for the body they have, not the body they could have. They settle for what others tell them is possible, not what they really want.

The problem with settle-itis is that once it infects one part of your life, it spreads like a cancer throughout every other aspect. You start to settle for a job you don't really like or a relationship you're not really happy in. You start living in the land of "good enough." And let me tell you something—once you move into that neighborhood, it *ain't* easy moving out.

I hate wasting time and money, and I was doing plenty of both. So after that Christmas, I told myself I had a choice: I could throw up my hands and say this is the body nature gave me, or I could use the brain God gave me and figure things out.

I decided to take control and figure things out. One weekend right after Christmas, I laid out the meal plans from every diet I had tried. Next to them I placed the countless workout plans I had followed, along with the countless fitness and nutrition books I had read. Then I filtered out what worked to some degree, what might work if I tweaked it, and what was useless. Through my own knowledge of physiology and more experimentation, I created a workout and nutrition plan that took me from having no muscle definition to having the body of my dreams.

I went from this:                    to this:

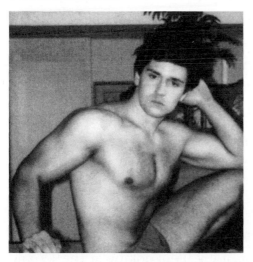 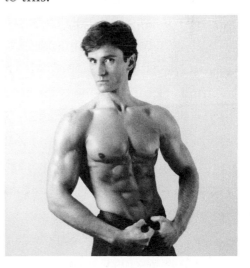

Not exactly a bar of soap anymore, huh?

# JOHN-ISM

If you dream it, you can do it.
Never give up on your dreams.

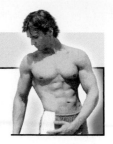

But here's the thing: it wasn't just my body that was transformed. I had energy and focus. I had goals, and I had reawakened the drive to achieve them. When I realized the miraculous improvements I made with the plan I devised, when I realized that I had the power to dramatically change something so basic as the body I thought I was stuck with, that empowered me and gave me the confidence to go after goals in other areas of my life as well. It had always been a dream of mine to model for a fitness magazine, and within a few months I turned that dream into a reality. In fact, I appeared in just about every exercise magazine on the market. I started thinking, "If my plan can do this for me, maybe it could help save other people wasted time, effort, and frustration in trying to get the bodies they want." I christened my plan Fitness Made Simple and decided to spread the word. I actually began to feel my goals were within my grasp.

I wanted to control my destiny this time. I took the experience and contacts I had developed from my "Images" television days and put together the first Fitness Made Simple video on a shoestring budget. Because I lacked the funds to hire anyone else—hell, I was still searching for loose change on the floor of my car—I had to become an expert in all aspects of the television business and print media to promote Fitness Made Simple. I wrote a column for a fitness magazine in exchange for advertising space. I called the TV stations for airtime and placed every one of my commercials nationwide by myself.

The first Fitness Made Simple commercial went on the air later that summer. It was the most magical moment of my life. Looking at the TV and seeing myself staring back—tears were about to come to my eyes. I had been on television before, of course, but this was different. This was such a personal victory. Before long the orders started coming in. I took customer service calls, I packed boxes on my parents' couch until 3 A.M., and then I carried those packages off to the post office every morning in a big Santa sack. "John," the postal workers would say, "we see your commercials at night, and then we see you bringing in the boxes in the morning!"

That was just the beginning. The commercials got better and better, and the videos had bigger and bigger budgets. Between August and December—only a few months—my life completely transformed. I started getting letters and cards from many, many people about how this one video had changed their lives. They had the bodies and lives they wanted. The phone rang so often that I found myself using a phony voice again—not to avoid bill collectors but because people loved the program so much they wanted to date me! It was an amazing accomplishment, a breakthrough moment for me.

Christmas came again, a year after the worst Christmas of my life.

I had driven to my parents' house from my place—*my* place, not the bank's. My aunt was on the phone again. She wanted to talk to me first.

"John."

Pause.

"I saw you on television. Can you send me some signed photos? No one believes I'm your aunt! Oh, and my friend wants me to ask you if I can get her an autograph. She's been on your program, and it's completely changed her life."

Just like it will change yours.

FITNESS MADE SIMPLE

The Fitness Made Simple program can change the bodies and lives of anyone from teenagers to grandparents. My lawyers tell me I have to say "results not typical" when I talk about the remarkable transformations people have

Dear John,

I am writing to thank you for your instruction on exercise and nutrition. As a teenager I was overweight and inactive. I have fought most of my adult life to keep weight off and stay fit. I spent 25 years jogging and 15 years working out at a gym four to five times a week with machines and free weights. I've also tried many popular diet plans, including fasting. None of these activities have given me the results that your program helped me to achieve in two short months. Fitness Made Simple helped me reach a physical fitness level that had eluded me all my life. I have lost 22 pounds, five inches off my waist, and five inches off my hips. I have dropped from a size 10 to a size 4 in slacks. My energy level is high and I really feel good about myself. FMS showed me how to work out efficiently and do the exercises correctly. It puts an emphasis on working the abs, an area that I had avoided. It also gave me the nutritional tips I needed that explained how I sabotaged myself in the past when trying to lose body fat. My husband, Fred, and I both enjoy cooking and, thanks to the

seen, but after getting letter upon letter telling me of 40 pounds dropped, 15 percent of body fat vanishing, or abs showing after a lifetime of trying, I start to wonder if these results *are* typical for Fitness Made Simple.

And here's the thing about the program: it changes your life, but it doesn't take over your life.

tips FMS provides, with very little effort
we were able to change our eating
habits to a healthful, fat-burning style.
I hate to call it a diet because to me
that word implies something painful that I will do for only
a short period of time. Since we changed our eating
habits we are never hungry and are enjoying very tasty
meals and snacks. The benefits are obvious and for us
this is a lifetime change.

My husband, Fred, who originally was skeptical, has reaped
a surprise benefit. In three months he has lost more than
40 pounds. He still has a way to go but is so encouraged that
he is confident of getting down to his "fighting weight." In addition,
after having observed the positive results I have obtained with
the exercises, he is now planning to follow the exercise program
as well.

Fitness Made Simple does bring real results to real people.
I am a grandmother and celebrated my 65th birthday this month.
My husband, Fred, is 67. Please keep up the good work.

You may have been expecting me to tell you that you'll have to spend hours a day in the gym or go on a diet prescribed by St. Benedict himself. But I believe that fitness is not a game of how miserable you can make yourself. It's not about torture, deprivation, and endless workouts. Your fitness routine should be something that you not only tolerate but enjoy and look forward to. Otherwise, you're not going to stick to it. Fitness Made Simple makes incorporating fitness into your lifestyle fun, convenient, and unbelievably fulfilling. If you get involved in workouts you don't enjoy or in yo-yo dieting, it's like handing yourself a "Fat for Life" card. If you try to follow a plan you hate, in eight weeks you'll have a Pop-Tart in one hand and the remote in the other.

Fitness Made Simple gives people great results because it works *with* human nature, not against it. It's not a short-term diet; it's a lifestyle change. I'll get into details starting in the next chapter, but right now I'll give you three basic ideas that make Fitness Made Simple work:

- Train smarter, not harder.
- Eat more, not less.
- Supplements are great as supplements, not as substitutes for an effective workout and nutrition program.

The program I created based on those three ideas has helped people from 18 to 80.

You're going to meet some of those FMS Success Stories throughout this book and read many of the letters and e-mails I've gotten, but here's one of my favorites. Her name is Elizabeth, and when she first started Fitness Made Simple she was a 64-year-old grandmother who had been waging a 50-year war with her weight. "I've been counting calories for half a century," she told me. She had tried plenty of exercise plans, but they had her working way too hard for way too few gains. Fitness Made Simple got her to train smarter, not harder. The result? Elizabeth now looks like she could win a fitness contest. "I have lost 22 pounds, five inches off my waist, and five inches off my hips. My clothes are falling off!" As great as Elizabeth looks now, the real miracle in that family is her husband, Fred. He's lost 40 pounds, gotten off his blood pressure medication, and taken himself out of medical danger.

I'd be pleased if Fitness Made Simple helps you lose a few pounds and feel better. That would be great, but I won't be satisfied.

I know—I'm living proof—fitness has a ripple effect that just makes everything better, physically, mentally, and emotionally. It is mediocrity's mortal enemy and the only cure I know for settle-itis. And the land of "good enough" I talked about earlier? Fitness Made Simple is your ticket out of that place. Fitness Made Simple helps you realize your power to be special, your power to stand out in a world that's trying to make you like everyone else.

In our cars, the windshield is big and open. The rearview mirror is tiny. That's because what's in front—the future—is important to us. The past, not so much. Look at what's in front of you and not toward what was good enough for you before. I'd love it if you changed your life with FMS. Once you take control of your body, it gives you the confidence to go after all of your other dreams as well.

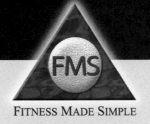

FITNESS MADE SIMPLE

# THE THREE STEPS TO FITNESS

If you're unhappy with how your body looks, you've probably tried a program or two to lose weight or build muscle. In fact, you may have tried a lot of programs and most of them didn't work. Is it your fault? I doubt it. Most people aren't lazy asses. They're intelligent, disciplined, and hard-working. But they fail when it comes to fitness because they're using the wrong knowledge. As I put it in one of the most popular John-isms, *trying to get in shape with the wrong knowledge is like trying to open a door with the wrong key.*

That's what Fitness Made Simple did for me and what it can do for you. It will give you the right key to unlock the door to fitness so that all your discipline, hard work, and dedication are put to good use.

Let's get back to those ill-fitting keys for a minute. Most of them don't work for a simple reason: they offer only a dumbed-down, one-dimensional approach to changing your body. The advertisers and marketers on Madison Avenue are great at this. A while back, they told us that the secret to a great body was not eating fat: *as soon as you don't eat fat, you'll have the body of your dreams!* Now I don't believe you should eat a *lot* of fat, but there are plenty of physiological reasons why a fat-free diet alone isn't going to make you lean—and may do just the opposite. That's exactly what happened. After a few years of eating less fat, Americans were still getting bigger and bigger because blood sugar and insulin levels were spiking, thanks to all those fat-free goodies. That's the perfect biological environment to maximize fat storage.

So Madison Avenue did what it always does. It changed its message. *You know, guys, we were wrong about fat. The real key is not eating carbs! Eating no carbs is the way to the body of your dreams!* Now I don't believe in a high-carb diet, but I also don't believe you should completely eliminate any macronutrient. It seems I've been proven right. Even on this newfangled extremely low-carb eating scheme, most Americans don't look much leaner to me.

I was as big a sucker for these weight-loss gimmicks as anyone. Remember back when I first tried to change my White Castle–gorging ways—and failed

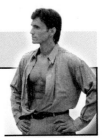

## JOHN-ISM

Reality is a self-imposed boundary created in people's minds so they can find solace in failure or comfort in not even trying.

miserably? Well, I tried a no-fat diet. And a no-carb diet. And just about every other get-a-great-body gimmick you can imagine. Here are a few that stand out (for how bad they were):

- **Bulking and cutting.** If you've spent much time in a gym, you've heard of this approach. The idea is to spend a few months bulking up by lifting weights, doing no cardio, and eating lots of calories and then cutting up by reducing calories. Let me tell you, in my opinion, it's the biggest fallacy in the world and basically just an excuse to find comfort in overeating. For starters, it seems like no one ever reaches the cutting stage. You see all these big guys gorging themselves during the winter in their "bulking phase," but then summer comes and they're still gorging! Even the guys who do cut up often don't see the results they were after. They somehow think the muscle fairy is going to preserve all the lean mass they built and only get rid of the fat. At least in my experience it doesn't happen that way in the real world.

  When I tried bulking and cutting, I only got fatter. My body was naturally shaped like a bowling pin narrow shoulders, long skinny arms, long skinny legs, and a big wide middle. When I bulked up, I just became a bigger bowling pin.

  So I moved on to . . .

- **The starvation approach,** also known as the world's oldest weight-loss plan. Want to drop pounds? Stop eating! Actually, in the beginning this can be rewarding. You're restricting calories and noticing yourself getting smaller. But you don't realize that your body is extremely smart, extremely adaptable, and it doesn't give a damn about how you look. It only wants to survive. When you restrict food, your body says, *OK, I don't know when this idiot is going to feed me next, so when he does I'm going to hold on to as much of that meal as I can.* Your metabolism slows down and you go into fat-storage mode. The minute you start eating normally again, you gain weight at a record rate.

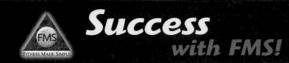
John,

I just wanted to let you know that your nutritional insights and training tips helped me achieve a body I never thought possible. I'm proud to say that I have dropped my body fat percentage from an unhealthy 23 percent to an unbelievable 7 percent, plus I've experienced gains in energy, strength, stamina, and endurance that are indescribable.

With the aid of your *Six Pack Abs* video, I've achieved the physique and positive mind-set I always wanted but was never able to achieve before. Anyway, I just thought I'd let you know that your work made a difference in my life and that I greatly appreciate what you have done for me and so many others.

You've probably seen people who've done this. They starve themselves for a few months, and you're thinking, *Hey, they look good.* But the next time you see them, they're looking a little too skinny—like I did when I tried this. When you see them six months later, after they've thrown in the towel and returned to their usual eating habits, they're fatter than ever before.

So that approach didn't work for me either. Is it any wonder I next tried . . .

- **The tuna and pineapple diet.** This was the most ridiculous thing I did. I ate tuna and pineapple every day for every single meal. The tuna was supposed to build muscle, and the pineapple killed the taste of the tuna. I don't think it put on any pounds, but it certainly didn't cut me up much. Worse, it just made me miserable. I didn't look forward to meals, and none of my friends wanted to eat with me. Can you blame them? I'd

The really cool thing is a lot of people are starting to get curious about FMS, along with health and nutrition in general. I'm getting asked a lot of questions, and I'm doing my best to answer them. I've been explaining the benefits of health and nutrition, never failing to mention how the FMS program has changed my life. Again, I'd like to thank you for providing the inspiration and knowledge that has helped make a great difference in my life.

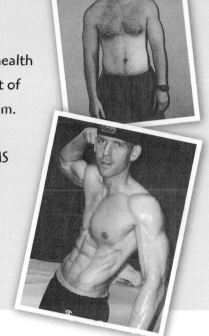

have my smelly little plastic tuna container and these ridiculous pineapple rings. It was also really annoying to have to carry a can opener wherever I went.

If you tried any of these diets or others like them, I can empathize. I know how frustrating it is to throw yourself into something and have it fail miserably.

After a year of doing all this stuff, I still didn't have any visible abs. I guess my body shape changed to some degree, but I couldn't see it because I still sported a significant layer of subcutaneous fat, which is the definition-obscuring flab between our skin and muscle layers. I wasn't obese, but I was somebody who had to defend the fact that I worked out.

"I go to the gym," I'd mention to someone.

## JOHN-ISM

Turn obstacles into opportunities. Transform problems into possibilities.

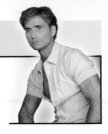

"You do?" they'd say, looking me up and down. I knew what they were thinking: *ain't nothing I'm seeing showing me that, John.*

I was getting nowhere near the return I should have received for my exercise investment. If you're going to spend X amount of time doing something, you want to get a return—at least I do. If you spend $100,000 on a college education, study every day, and all of a sudden the dean says you're not going to graduate, then you'd be pretty pissed, wouldn't you? Well, I was pissed.

Then came that fateful Christmas. When I sat down the following weekend to look hard at what I'd been doing, I realized that no single thing was going to get me in great shape. There was no miracle diet or revolutionary workout. There were no magic pills or potions. I knew I needed something more than a one-dimensional approach. I needed something that combined nutrition, exercise, and supplements.

As it turned out, that was the key to open the door.

## LOOKING AT FITNESS WITH 3-D GLASSES

The Fitness Made Simple plan is based on a triangle. The first side is nutrition. The second side is exercise. The third side is proper supplementation. All three sides of the triangle are important, but they're not all equal.

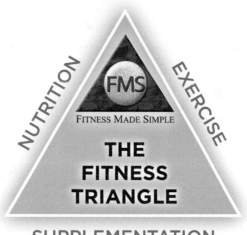

Building your body is like building a house. The nutrition and exercise sides of the triangle are your foundation and walls. The supplement side represents your accessories, furniture, decorations, and paintings. You can't hang a painting without first erecting a wall. As I said earlier, there are no magic pills and potions. If you don't have an effective fitness foundation—meaning a solid workout and nutrition plan—most supplements will have little to no effect on improving your physique. However, if you do have that foundation, an effective supplement will do wonders for maximizing your results.

I'll give you the details of each side of the triangle in future chapters. Right now, let me touch on the basics.

## Nutrition: Eat More, Not Less

Your workouts will make your muscles grow, but your eating habits will make them show. I believe proper nutrition is more important than any other aspect when it comes to building your ultimate physique.

That, however, doesn't mean you're going on a diet. I hate the word *diet*. Diets suck. Diets make you think of deprivation, and life's too short for deprivation. That's why the phrase I use is *nutrition plan*.

The FMS nutrition plan is based on two ideas. First, *eat four to six small meals a day*. That's right, I want you to eat more often, not less often. Eating six meals is actually best, but you can get away with four or five meals since I've seen good results with these numbers as well. Four to six small, balanced meals a day keep your body happy and your energy up. Eating this way decreases cravings that lead to fattening snacks and helps you stay in a steady, fat-burning mode throughout the day.

The other key idea is to *mix all three macronutrients—fats, proteins, and carbohydrates—at every meal.* Good fats, like the poly- and monounsaturated kind, are essential for everything from preventing heart disease to having great skin. Protein is crucial for building muscle. Slow-burning carbohydrates give you long-lasting energy that keeps you from feeling run-down or hungry. That's why I want you to *think "F-M-S" at every meal. F* stands for "Fantastic Fats." *M* stands for "Muscle-Maximizing Proteins." *S* stands for "Slow-Burning Carbs." You should have a combination of them all at every meal.

## Exercise: Train Smarter, Not Harder

You don't have to spend hours a day in the weight room to get the body you've been dreaming of. In fact, when it comes to fitness, *more is not always better.* I know this firsthand. One of the biggest mistakes I made was overtraining. I worked out with weights six or seven days a week and didn't give my body a chance to rest. Muscles grow during *rest* periods. You break down muscle fibers during workouts, stimulating them to regrow bigger and stronger with the help of proper nutrition and adequate rest. Back in the day I left out that last part of the equation, so I ended up overtraining my body, which led to a whole host of other problems.

Weight training is essential, but the key words should be *short* and *intense.* Under my plan you'll lift weights only every other day (three or four times per week) and for no more than an hour at a time. You also don't need to worry about joining a gym because most of the exercises I recommend can be done at home with a basic set of adjustable dumbbells and an inexpensive bench.

Another component of the Fitness Made Simple workout plan is *morning cardio.* Blood-sugar and insulin levels are lowest in the morning, when your stomach is empty. That's the perfect environment for burning fat. I'll share a little secret with you: nothing else I did—no pill, potion, or nutrition plan—made a bigger difference when it came to fat loss than when I started to do my cardio in the morning before my first meal.

## Supplements: They're Great as Supplements, Not as Substitutes

Unless you already have the basic building blocks for an effective workout and meal plan in place, I don't really recommend jumping on the heavily advertised supplement bandwagon. Here's another John-ism for you: *supplements are not substitutes for sound exercise and eating.*

That said, once the other two sides of the triangle are in place, the addition of an effective fat-burning or muscle-building supplement can help speed and maximize the results of your gym and kitchen efforts. They're also great for renewing your enthusiasm and overcoming plateaus in a fitness routine.

Fair warning: there's a lot of hype out there when it comes to supplements, and most supplements aren't worth the money you spend on them. I'll go over which supplements have been the most beneficial for me in delivering cosmetically significant results when it comes to building muscle and losing fat.

# THE BENEFITS OF FITNESS

So those are the basics of the program. Throughout the rest of the book, I'm going to show you how to implement them into your day, so that you really change your body and life for good.

The changes can be amazing, and they go way beyond the cosmetic ones like having a six-pack at the beach or fitting into a particular dress size.

Dear FMS,

I'm 36 years old, I'm in the best shape of my life, and my shape is getting better every day, thanks to Fitness Made Simple. I'm at this point because through FMS I finally got it. In order to make real improvements in my body, I had to combine changes in my diet, weight training, and cardio workouts. What a difference combining those three made!

I initially chose Fitness Made Simple because I was motivated by John's success story—how he changed his own body through the very same exercises I would be doing. Now I look forward to working out with John every day because he keeps me motivated and committed to the exercise programs. I have stuck with the programs because the exercises and the nutritional tips work! I notice the difference in my body and in how my clothes fit. These days I am wearing the tailored,

A lean, muscular body increases your metabolism since muscle is a fat-burning furnace. It increases resistance to many illnesses including heart disease, diabetes, and many cancers and helps you stay healthy. It increases your energy, self-esteem, and confidence, all of which then empower you to accomplish goals in other parts of your life. Following a fitness lifestyle simply improves everything—physically, mentally, and emotionally.

I won't lie to you or insult your intelligence by telling you it's going to be easy. Simple, yes, because the whole blueprint for improving your body will be laid out in future chapters, but you're still going to have to show commitment and dedication to achieve results. Some people who first hear my program say, "Ooh, that's going to be so difficult." Yeah, making important changes in your life *is* difficult. People who achieve great things have done difficult things.

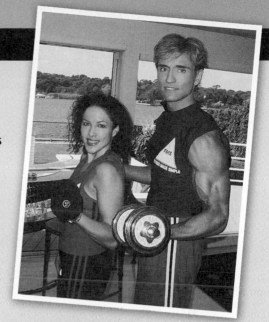

sexy clothes I love to wear, including sleeveless shirts. I just love the muscle tone I see all over my body.

What I have found to be particularly useful is John's tip that all I have to do is work on making one aspect of my routine better each day. Honestly, for me, it may take a few days to make my routine better, but it's OK because I realize that I am making changes for the rest of my life and not just for next week or month!

My body feels great, I feel great, and I have more energy than I have ever had—energy that comes in handy at Harvard Law School.

But here's the truth: difficulty fades with time. You're not going to remember how tough every day was when you're looking at the body of your dreams staring back at you in the bathroom mirror every day.

In the end, your benefits will be more than worth the effort. Starting a fitness lifestyle is the best investment you could ever make in yourself. The rewards you reap will change your world.

## JOHN-ISM

Bring people up to your level.
Don't sink to theirs.

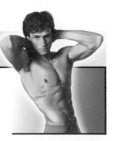

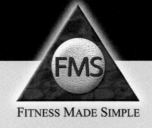

FITNESS MADE SIMPLE

# CHAPTER 3

# MY TOP 10 TIPS FOR LIVING LEAN AND HEALTHY

In upcoming chapters I'm going to go more in-depth on each side of the fitness triangle and give you specific, day-by-day programs you can follow to achieve the body of your dreams.

I know from experience, however, the reality of the situation. There are some days it's hard to stick to a detailed plan. That's why I came up with my Top 10 Tips for Living Lean and Healthy. Each of these tips helped me more than I can say, and they'll help you, too. They'll let you navigate your way through trying times or difficult situations. As with everything in the Fitness Made Simple program, I learned these strategies by living them. Some deal with the physical components of fitness—nutrition and exercise—while others focus on the mental aspect, which I believe is responsible for more than 50 percent of success in the fitness game, not to mention other aspects of your life.

Fitness begins in the mind. If you think it, you can do it. Think positively, and you can accomplish anything.

## 1. TAKE BABY STEPS

The words *baby steps* refer to the mind-set you should have when following a fitness lifestyle, especially when you're first starting out. Too many people think the only way they'll be successful and get the body they want is if they do everything all at once—exercise every day or go from fast-food burgers and fries to chicken breast and vegetables overnight. Just thinking about these drastic changes is overwhelming, and it causes most people to throw up their hands and quit their fitness programs before they even get started.

Instead, you should look at fitness as a lifelong journey and make an effort to think of improving one thing or doing one thing better fitness-wise each day. Do that every morning when you wake up, and by the end of a month you'll be 30 times better. One day you may say, "I'm going

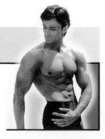

## JOHN-ISM
The only way to lose is if you quit.
Success doesn't have a time limit.

to do 100 stomach crunches today." Be specific. The next day you might look at your diet and eliminate one or two high-fat, high-sugar foods you normally eat. Then the day after that you may decide to start doing some of the yoga stretches I'll go over in the workout chapter. The specifics don't matter. *What matters is that you improve yourself and your fitness program each and every day.* When you do that it becomes self-motivating. You see the positive changes and you want more, and things that would have seemed impossible at the beginning of the month will now seem easy and natural.

## 2. EAT UNTIL YOU'RE NO LONGER HUNGRY, NOT FULL

There is a very fine distinction between feeling not hungry and feeling full, and it took me a while to learn to notice it. To avoid overeating you want to leave the table when you no longer feel hungry, when the food is beginning to not taste as good as it did originally and you're just continuing to eat it because it's there. You don't want to wait until you feel full. There's a biological reason for this. It takes the brain about 15 to 20 minutes before it realizes that the stomach is full, and then it sends the message to stop eating. That 15- to 20-minute lag time is what keeps a lot of extra pounds on our trouble-prone areas—the belly and lower back in men and the waist, hips, and thighs in women.

If you stop eating when you're no longer hungry, in about 15 to 20 minutes you will feel full. I know I do. If I wait until I actually feel full before leaving the table, in about 15 to 20 minutes it's couch time for me. I feel really bloated and tired and just want to lie down for a long nap. This is a big sign that you've overeaten and that you've overwhelmed your body's digestive process with the food intake. It doesn't have energy left over to do anything other than try to handle the food overload, so it signals you to take a rest.

You shouldn't feel exhausted after eating. Food is supposed to energize us. Since I learned how to tell the difference between being no longer hungry and feeling full, I have to say it works. I feel so much better after eating, and maintaining a lean weight is a lot easier.

# 3. DON'T STARVE AND STUFF

Starving is probably the worst thing most people do when trying to lose fat, and it sends the worst messages to our bodies.

1. Starving ourselves or depriving our bodies of food sends them into fat-storage mode, which is something no one wants. Our bodies are designed not to care how we look but to preserve our lives. When we starve them, they try to hold on to every last bit of fat reserves they have and fat burning just about stops. When we do finally eat again, we usually overeat and stuff ourselves, which really defeats our weight-loss efforts since our bodies are now primed to store as much of that feast as fat as they can get away with, much more than they would have stored if we just continued eating normally.

2. A starvation-type diet also causes the body, which is trying to preserve fat stores, to start catabolizing, or breaking down, other tissues like muscle, which is metabolically active and burns fat for energy. During a starvation situation muscle is the enemy. It's burning precious fat that the body wants to hold on to, so it's gotta go. When you start

eating normally again, you'll put on fat in record time, probably more than you ever had before, because you have less muscle mass to burn fat on a daily basis. In short, you've blunted your body's fat-burning capacity.

3. Finally, starving and stuffing creates emotional and mental turmoil. No one really wants to live like that.

# 4. DO A.M. CARDIO

Doing cardio first thing in the A.M. is our fat cells' worst nightmare. It's the best time for burning body fat. In the morning, after a good night's sleep and before we eat, our bodies are going to burn a greater percentage of stored body fat for energy rather than relying on energy from food we've just eaten. Our blood-sugar and insulin levels are low and stable, which is the perfect environment for fat burning to occur. After we eat, especially after we eat meals high in carbs, our blood-sugar and insulin levels rise and fat burning stops.

When I first added morning cardio to my fitness routine, I started dropping pounds of fat like a bad habit. If your schedule doesn't permit you to do cardio first thing in the morning, you can add it after your workout or later at night. But try to make sure it's done on an empty stomach. For variety you can use a treadmill, stair-climber, elliptical trainer, or stationary bike, or you can simply walk, jog, or run around the block a few times. I just make sure to keep it low impact so my heart rate stays in fat-burning mode. If you're huffing and puffing, you're probably working too hard and possibly breaking down muscle tissue. You should be able to carry on a conversation without losing your breath.

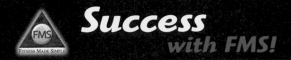

Hello John,

Thank you, thank you, thank you. My work-out is a consistent on/off FMS, cardio, FMS, cardio—using your *Six Pack Abs* workout on my cardio days. It's been about eight weeks and I have a completely different body doing this and using your nutrition tips. Your words stand true. Not only has FMS changed my body, but it has changed my mind as well. I feel like I can accomplish anything by applying your philosophy.

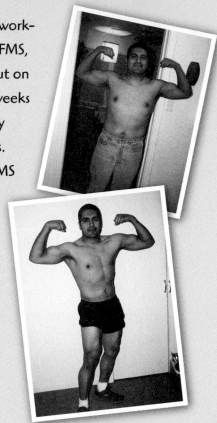

**MY STATS:** 33 years old, 5'10"
**START:** 210 pounds, tight 34-inch waist pant size
**EIGHT WEEKS:** 195 pounds, 31-inch waist pant size

I have seen considerable changes all over, with my legs being the most apparent. Again, thank you, thank you, thank you!

# 5. DRINK WATER

Water is a magical drink. It helps transport vitamins, minerals, and other nutrients throughout our bodies, plus it flushes out toxins and other waste products. Our muscles consist of 70 percent water, so drinking lots of it helps keep them looking full and pumped.

I like to drink lots of water, about a gallon a day, not only for its health benefits but also because it helps keep me lean. I drink it with and in between meals to curb my appetite and decrease cravings. I also learned another trick to stop overeating: if I'm getting ready for a photo shoot or personal appearance, I'll have a full 8- to 10-ounce glass of water *before* each meal starting a few days prior to the event. I noticed it fills up my stomach and causes me to eat much less than I normally would if I didn't down the water first. Water's my best friend when it comes to sticking to a lower-calorie nutrition plan.

# 6. BE A SMART SHOPPER

My sixth tip for living lean and healthy relates to shopping. We all do it, but we don't all do it well. Be a smart shopper.

First off, *don't ever go food shopping when you're hungry*. Your stomach will always override your brain. Cravings kick common sense to the curb, and you'll end up with a cart full of sugar- and saturated-fat-filled garbage that you bought on impulse rather than planning.

Second, *don't ever enter the supermarket without a list*—and don't buy anything other than what's on that list, especially when you're first starting a new nutrition plan or fitness program. Think before you put something on your list about what benefit it will bring you and whether or not it will help or hinder you in achieving your fitness goals.

TAKE CONTROL OF YOUR BODY

Third, *try to shop in the outer aisles of the supermarket.* Along the periphery of the store is where you'll find more of the natural foods—vegetables, fruits, and protein sources like chicken breasts, turkey breasts, and egg whites. It's when you venture into those inner aisles that you get into trouble. That's where all the highly processed, high-calorie/high-carb/high-sugar nasties are. In general, the more highly processed a food is, the bigger the blood-sugar reaction it's going to give you and the further it's going to put you from attaining your fitness goals. Stick with natural choices. Save these inner aisles for last when you just want to get a treat or "cheat food" that you've been craving, or avoid them altogether.

## 7. MAKE BETTER "BAD" CHOICES

Now that we know how to shop, let's stick with the nutrition theme. Fitness is supposed to be fun, and eating healthy will actually be more fun than eating poorly. Our bodies crave what they're used to—the stuff we've been feeding them over time. If you subsist on fast-food hamburgers, milk shakes, and large brownies, like I used to, then that's what your body is living on and that's what it will crave. These cravings will change when you start feeding your body something different. When I first heard that I didn't believe it either. I thought I was born to crave bacon double cheeseburgers and jumbo fries, but I can tell you now that I wasn't. I don't even want them anymore. The problem is that it usually takes four to eight weeks for our bodies to get over old cravings and start craving the new, better foods. It's like lag time. We might want to look and feel better now, but our bodies want the sugar and saturated fat they've been surviving on so they don't react as quickly as we might like. During that time it helps to make better "bad" choices.

For example, if you crave ice cream, follow tip 1, take baby steps. Don't make yourself miserable by eliminating it altogether; instead, eat it a little less frequently or have a smaller portion than you normally would—or choose a more waistline-friendly alternative like sugar-free, fat-free frozen yogurt. If you crave tacos, try a "better" alternative like what I call Fitness Made Simple Chicken Wraps, which have all the basic ingredients of a chicken taco except the deep-fried, saturated-fat-filled tortilla shell. That's where most of the calories and fat grams are. Instead, I wrap the chicken and vegetables in a lettuce shell, which adds next to no calories. You can still dip this creation in your favorite sauces and it will taste great, plus you won't feel guilty later, like you cheated on your meal plan.

I've learned you sometimes have to play little mental games to break bad habits while you're trying to set good ones in motion. One of the tricks I came up with I call "Natural Days." When I was trying to break out of my fast-food, pizza, and chocolate diet and get leaner, every other or every third day I would make a Natural Day, where I'd eat only natural foods: raw vegetables, a few fruits, protein sources like chicken breast, and nuts like almonds or all-natural peanut butter for "good" fat. It was like going through detox, but it worked. The protein and vegetables really filled me up, decreased my cravings for the junk, and helped me get leaner more quickly.

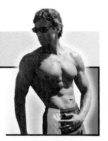

## JOHN-ISM

Excuses are like armpits: everybody has them and most stink. Believe in yourself and don't let anything stand in the way of attaining your dreams.

Dear John,

My name is Jason McMurray and I am a 21-year-old male living in Santa Cruz, California. In high school I had always managed to stay in shape because I was constantly training for track and cross-country all year-round, running on average 10 miles a day. A few years ago I moved up here to Santa Cruz for college, excited for my independence. Because there was no great sports program at my school, I was not active on any teams and did not get nearly as much exercise as my body was used to from four years of running. As a result I gained a bit more than the normal "freshman 15" and was not happy with how quickly my body was looking less healthy. I knew something needed to change.

I then started on your Fitness Made Simple program and have been following it for more than a year now. I've seen an amazing amount of improvement in my body and health. I feel and look better than I ever have in my life!

FMS not only has given me a much healthier lifestyle but has made a dramatic improvement in my ability to train for my profession. I am

# 8. KEEP "CHEAT" FOODS OUT OF THE HOUSE

Cheating can be a good thing. It's fun and it can also be guilt-free. As long as we exercise regularly and eat clean the majority of the day, having a bite or two of something we've been craving is generally going to have no an ex-UCSC student currently studying to become a paramedic and firefighter. Both of these jobs are very physical so the vast improvements I made in my exercise habits and diet have given me the energy I need to make it through every day feeling great.

Although your workout plan proved very effective for me in the gym, the nutritional tips really helped make the most drastic improvements in my body. FMS has inspired in me a passion for health and fitness, and I'm currently in a 12-week course to receive my ACE Personal Trainer Certification. I owe it all to the inspiration and guidance I have received from your program.

I cannot thank you enough for the kindness and inspiration you've shown me. I only hope that everyone will eventually realize they *can* take control over their own lives, which is something you helped me to see.

noticeable or visible impact on the lean physique we're trying to build, plus it will help us keep our sanity.

There's only one rule I follow when it comes to cheating: keep "cheat" foods out the house. I know if I had brownies or anything with dark chocolate and nuts in my refrigerator, I'd probably never see my abs again. If, however, I want a brownie but I have to go to the local bakery or supermarket

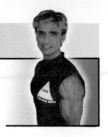

## JOHN-ISM

Don't be an energy vacuum,
sucking the joy from people.
Negative people can clear a room
quicker than a fart.

to get one, that's a totally different story. A craving is generally an impulse thing; it's usually satisfied without much thought and then we feel guilty later. If I have to go out to satisfy my craving, it gives me a moment to consider if it's really worth the trip. Once I think about the effort needed to get in the car, drive to the store, buy the brownie, and then go home and eat it, I generally find it's not worth the trouble and the urge passes. It sounds funny but it works. It's all about having conscious thought take control over impulse. Keeping cheat foods at home within arm's reach is just too tempting and sets us up for failure.

## 9. VARY EXERCISE CHOICES

To keep your body guessing and continue to stimulate growth, vary your exercise choices. As with anything done over time, our bodies and minds get used to certain workouts, causing us to reach a plateau where we stop seeing the same benefits from our exercise investments. That's usually because both our bodies and minds have become bored with the routine. They've been through it day in and day out, they know what to expect, and they've adjusted. To avoid getting stuck in an exercise rut, keep things fresh both mentally and physically by mixing and matching different workouts. I'll give you some options in later chapters. Changing workouts on a weekly or monthly basis really helps me maximize results.

# 10. THINK—AND THINK POSITIVELY

The one common thread that ties the mental, physical, and nutritional aspects together when we're trying to improve our fitness is thought—conscious thought, not acting on impulse or out of habit. Too many people, myself included, fall into the trap of just doing the same things day in and day out—I call it "sleepwalking" through life—and then complaining or finding excuses about why their bodies or lives aren't better.

Bottom line: a large part of how you look and feel today is a sum total of what you've been doing up to this point, so if you don't change what you're doing, you'll keep looking and feeling how you do right now. If you're happy with how you are now, then that's great; otherwise, it's time to start taking control of your life and your body and stop sleepwalking. Think about everything you do each day—what you eat, how much activity you get, and so on—and start making changes for the better, no excuses.

One of the first changes I made was to start thinking positively. Believe in yourself and you can accomplish anything. You achieve what you believe. If you can't envision yourself with a great body living a great life, you'll probably never get there, but if you keep that image in your head every day and work hard to achieve it, you'll probably be surprised by how quickly it turns into reality.

# THE
# FITNESS
# TRIANGLE

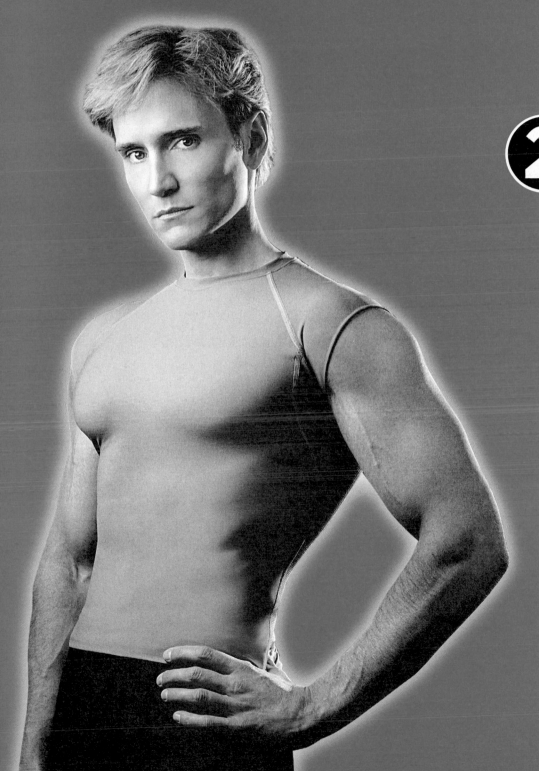

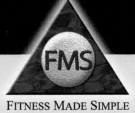

FITNESS MADE SIMPLE

# NUTRITION
## MADE
## SIMPLE

I said it before and I'll say it again: I believe that nutrition is the most important part of any fitness program. You're not going to look like a sleekly defined racehorse if you're eating like a pig.

And let's get rid of the excuses right now: eating well takes no more time or money than eating poorly. All it takes is the proper knowledge—the right key to open the door to a fantastic body.

No matter if you're trying to get that great look of leanness with eye-popping six-pack abs or if you're parading around 10, 20, even 50 pounds heavier than you'd like to be, your nutrition goal should be the same: to build muscle and lose fat. For those of you who are trying to get in shape after a period of being uncomfortably large, this means dropping pounds of goop on your thighs, middle, butt, or even (and you know who you are) the underside of your arms. Others of you may be trying to drop the last few pounds that stand between you and your aesthetic goal, meaning that stubborn layer of sub- cutaneous body fat lying between your skin and muscle, which obscures definition. As I know well, this can be a very difficult thing to do, espe- cially considering all of the contradictory and misleading nutrition advice around today. The diets du jour—the fat-free, carb-free, brain-free media hype we're bombarded with—do nothing but confuse us. Meanwhile, America is getting fatter every day.

That's why you're not going to go on a "diet." Not only do diets imply deprivation, but the scientific truth is that most traditional diets fail. They lead the dieter into the yo-yo syndrome of gaining and losing weight over and over again. This practice can be very unhealthy, to say the least. Diets also imply short-term goals, and most dieters stick to their diets for only a limited amount of time. That's why I like to think of my nutrition regimen as a nutrition plan—a plan that's a lifelong journey, not an overnight trip. Along this journey there will be good days when you eat well and travel a smooth road. There will also be detours and stopovers where you may cheat and succumb to cravings, after which you just get right back on the road to good eating again.

## JOHN-ISM

The challenge is to be yourself in a world that's trying to make you be like everyone else.

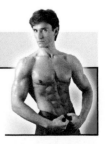

Back in my hamburger-eating lard-ass days, I was clueless about how my body processed the foods I ate. I tried many different diets and fads but still couldn't see my abs, even when I trained them every day. After filtering out the garbage that didn't work for me, I was able to come up with a few rules of basic nutrition that, for me, provided clarity in a world of confusion. These rules helped me work *with* my body, not *against* it, when it came to building muscle and losing fat.

They were the keys that let me open the door to achieving, in eight weeks, the muscular definition—including that tight six-pack of cut abs—I'd been working more than a year to get.

# THE BASICS

I'll lay out those rules of eating in a minute. First, we need to cover some basics that will help you understand the plan as well as, I hope, give you the knowledge and control you need to change your body—and your life—for good.

Food is divided into three basic groups: proteins, carbohydrates, and fats. These are known as the macronutrients. Contrary to popular belief, none of these macronutrients, not even fat, is inherently evil. In fact, I make sure to have some of each every day—ideally, at every meal. Here's why:

## Protein

Protein is nature's best muscle builder and also one of its best fat-loss aids. That's because it's the macronutrient least likely to be converted into body fat. It's the most metabolically costly for our bodies to process; thus it helps to increase our metabolism. Just as important, protein is a potent appetite suppressant and helps to decrease cravings throughout the day. In one major study, people who ate a morning meal made up of 50 percent protein *ate 25 percent fewer calories throughout the day.*

Good protein sources include chicken breast, turkey breast, fish, lean cuts of red meat, egg whites, tofu, lentils, and whey protein powders. I suggest limiting your intake of calorie-rich, fat-laden protein sources such as fatty meats, whole dairy products, and whole eggs.

## Carbohydrates

Carbs give us energy. Without them we'd have trouble making it through our day—or at least I did. When I went on an extreme low-carb diet, I got up around noon, needed a nap by three o'clock, had no energy to exercise, and just felt spacey all day long.

Carbohydrates are divided into two groups: high glycemic (high GI) carbs and low glycemic (low GI) carbs. Trust me, the two groups are not created equal. High GI carbs cause a rapid rise in blood-sugar levels, which in turn causes a rapid rise in insulin to "mop up" all that excess blood sugar and shuttle it into cells. Why is this a problem? Well, whatever is not shuttled into muscle cells, used for energy, or excreted as waste is stored as body fat. The more high GI carbs you ingest, the more likely you are to pack on the pounds.

High GI foods are usually the highly processed goodies that so many of us crave: sugary drinks and fruit juices, "junk" cereals, fat-free cookies, and that unwary dieter's favorite, the rice cake. Most of these foods not only cause water retention and bloat you, but they also interfere with your body's ability to tap into stored fat for energy, again making you more likely to gain weight. Believe it or not, the situation gets even worse. These processed foods also cause energy highs and lows as well as mood swings.

Low GI carbs, on the other hand, don't cause this rapid rise in blood sugar or the insulin spike that can lead to weight gain. Your body processes them more evenly over time, and they give you longer-lasting energy. Low GI carbohydrates include vegetables, sweet potatoes, 100 percent whole-grain breads, and my favorite, all-natural oatmeal.

## GLYCEMIC INDEX OF FOODS

The lower the glycemic index (GI) of a food, the slower and usually more desirable the blood-sugar response. In general, natural complex carbohydrates, such as oatmeal and yams, cause a more steady release of energy, whereas simple sugar and highly processed foods, such as white bread and rice cakes, cause a more rapid blood-sugar response, which leads to the all-too-common insulin surge that can result in unwanted fat storage. If you're planning to do a lot of exercise, high GI foods will provide instant energy, but if you don't use all of this energy, you can fall victim to rapid peaks and drops in blood-sugar levels, which can lead to feelings of moodiness, fatigue, and intense cravings.

Eating high GI foods, such as rice cakes, in combination with more slowly digested foods, such as fats, proteins, or lower GI carbohydrates, will help to level your blood-sugar response. That's why the Fitness Made Simple nutrition plan advises to always eat foods in combination. Rice cakes, for instance, are an acceptable low-calorie carb addition to your meals as long as you eat them in combination with something that slows their breakdown and absorption, such as the good monounsaturated-fat, all-natural peanut butter.

## Fat

Many of us have been repeatedly lied to when we're told that fat is inherently evil and bad for us. In my opinion, nothing could be further from the truth.

We're just beginning to wake up from this dietary catastrophe, but much of the damage has already been done. During the fat-free craze, I only noticed people increasing in weight. Many of the products on store shelves still advertise themselves as fat-free while being loaded with high

GI substitutions to make them palatable. In most cases it would be far better for our waistlines if we just ate the fat.

For me, fat is a key component of any nutrition plan due to the many benefits it provides. Fat lowers the glycemic index of foods, improves insulin resistance, maintains healthy skin and hair, protects neurological function, enables hormone production (especially key muscle-building hormones), and empowers fat metabolism.

That being said, I do want to point out that not all natural fats are created equal, meaning there are both "good" and "bad" fats. The first group of good fat is essential polyunsaturated fatty acids, which our bodies cannot make, so they must be obtained from food sources. My favorite is flaxseed oil. Flaxseed oil helps to block fat storage, increase metabolism, and increase insulin sensitivity. In some cases, it has been shown to be anti-catabolic. In other words, it helps stop muscle tissue breakdown. The other group of good fats is monounsaturated fats, like all-natural peanut butter, olive oil, and avocados.

The bad fats are saturated fats, which are primarily present in fatty meats, full-fat dairy products, and some tropical oils. Then there are trans-fatty acids. These processed wonder molecules give foods—especially baked goods—shelf stability and enduring "freshness," if something three months old in plastic can really be called fresh at all. While trans fats are great for keeping products sellable, they're terrible at keeping you alive. Trans fats are implicated in all manner of diseases, most notably heart disease. Thankfully, new labeling laws mandate that trans fats be listed on the labels of all processed foods. If possible, avoid them entirely. They don't occur in nature. When it comes to nutrition, I prefer to stick with *natural* choices. If it's made by man, you don't necessarily want to put it in your mouth.

In a typical day, I recommend that one-third of your fats come from the essential polyunsaturated fatty acids group, one-third from the mono-unsaturated fats group, and no more than one-third from the saturated

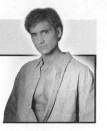

## JOHN-ISM

Don't tell me what I should do until you show me what you can do.

fats group. Saturated fat is almost impossible to avoid, since there are trace amounts present in many of the otherwise beneficial foods we eat.

# MY FIVE SIMPLE RULES FOR GOOD NUTRITION

With this major knowledge in place, it's time to delve into your nutrition plan. It's the same plan that took me from my old average self to the lean "Fitness Celebrity" that you see on TV—in just eight weeks! No matter what your goals are, this plan will get you there. If you've got a great deal of extra fat to lose, you'll probably need more than just eight weeks, but I promise you that if you follow this plan, you will be amazed by the positive changes it creates.

## 1. Have Four to Six Small, Balanced Meals a Day— Every Day

Eating four to six small, balanced meals a day, meaning every three to four hours, fights hunger and prevents you from cheating with fattening between-meal snacks. It also keeps your metabolism and energy levels high throughout the day. Our bodies are being trained to stay in a constant food-burning mode with a steady but not overwhelming flow of nutrients.

With only two to three large meals a day, your body gets overwhelmed from the relatively large amount of food it takes in at one time. Whatever

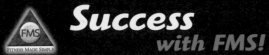

John,

I had to finally sit down and put into words the results I am getting with your program. I had lost a lot of weight, 80-plus pounds in a little over a year, using various diets and several exercise programs. I then hit a plateau. While I was no longer 222 pounds, I still wasn't anywhere near my goal.

I decided it was time to join a gym and lift weights since that was the one method I had not yet tried. For five months I worked out at the gym two hours a day, six to seven days a week, but my results were minimal. I had seen Fitness Made Simple commercials prior to this but never thought that someone with your body could ever understand a weight problem. I also assumed you had to be doing some crazy training that I could never get involved with because I have two small children at home and not a whole lot of time. Fortunately for me, you go to my gym and, over my five months of inefficient training, I watched you work out during my rest periods. That is what first interested me in your program. Your workout was less than half the duration of mine. It used to burn me up to see you walk in 20 minutes after me and leave 45 minutes before me. That's when I had to know what you were really doing so I ordered the basic FMS program.

Not only did I go from a size 10 to an 8 during the first three weeks of using Fitness Made Simple, but for the first time in months I started to see my strength really increase. I've actually doubled the weight I lift in some exercises in just three weeks! More amazing to me was that I was now only weight training three days a week for one hour as opposed to the ridiculous amount of time I was spending before and getting nowhere.

I used to use the excuse that my kids get up early and I had to feed them right away, blah, blah, blah. But your workout is so fast, and, because I use the nonweight version, the kids can be right there with me. I have done crunches with my son lying on top of me. My daughter likes to do push-ups so it works out and gets my metabolism going. I was spending 20 to 30 minutes every single day doing 500 to 600 useless incorrect sit-ups. Now I spend 10 minutes doing abdominal exercises that I actually feel and can see results with in only two weeks!

Overall, it has been five weeks and *I'm happy to say I am now a size 6!* I still have a bit to go but I know and can feel that I will get there using this system.

Thank you so much for creating it and doing all the legwork, research, and trial and error for me and everyone else who buys your products. You have saved others and me years of useless training because you didn't want people to go through what you did when you first got started and I think that is awesome. And for me personally, thanks for all your time in helping me understand things when I ask and for giving me different ideas and just listening. You truly care about the results people are getting and, from reading the testimonials of others you've helped, I know you are truly dedicated to working with anyone who is serious about changing his or her body and health. You are such a genuine person—real and giving—and you deserve so many great things for all that you are doing in the area of fitness for all the people out there who are benefiting from your hard work.

Thanks, John!

the body can't use at the time gets stored as—you guessed it—fat. Remember, anything that is not used by our bodies for energy or excreted as waste will be stored as fat for use later.

Eating by the clock will take some discipline and it will require you to take some food to work. However, you'll find it to be a simple adjustment, and your wallet will also thank you. Bringing some food from home is a heck of a lot cheaper than those saturated-fat, sugar-filled, and calorie-laden fast-food lunches we've all fallen victim to. By simply eating four to six small, balanced meals a day, you'll satiate your hunger, you won't feel like you're starving yourself, and you'll be raising your metabolism so that you burn more fat than you ever thought possible.

## 2. Watch Those Carbs

Unlike protein, which we now know dramatically decreases our cravings, carbohydrates, especially those simple carbs, have been shown to dramatically increase our appetites.

We experience a big blood-sugar surge when our meals are primarily carbohydrates and hardly any protein or fat. This rise in blood sugar often causes mood swings, and the subsequent rapid drop in blood sugar leads to a lethargic feeling that makes many high-carb eaters just want to take a nap. Even worse, when our body's energy reserves or glycogen stores are filled with carbs, the majority of the extra blood sugar floating around just gets converted to body fat. Carbs are our bodies' preferred fuel source. As long as we continue eating a lot of them, our bodies *won't* tap into fat stores at all. Why should they? They have all those carbs floating around. Burning body fat for energy happens when blood sugar is low.

Eating a diet too high in carbs can also lead to that bloated appearance since excess carbs tend to cause water retention. That's why some of the high-carb proponents have a sort of puffy look and aren't as toned and defined as their diets would suggest.

Excess dietary carbohydrates can lead to a chronically high insulin level. That, in turn, can cause insulin resistance, high cortisol levels, and, possibly, type 2 diabetes. Cortisol is a catabolic hormone—it breaks down muscle and other tissues. It is the enemy of a lean body. Moreover, high insulin levels are antagonistic to testosterone and growth hormone production. Those two substances are the body's best muscle-building hormones. That's why I maintain that food is only as relevant as the hormonal and biochemical pathways it affects. If you stay on a high-carbohydrate diet, you can go to the gym, work harder, and still remain a whole lot fatter.

By the way, the reason for those cravings is an evil little hormone called neuropeptide y. It signals the brain to crave more carbohydrates, and high GI dietary carbohydrates trigger this devil. Protein and fats don't. In other words, high GI carbohydrates signal the body to want *more* carbs.

So to keep your cravings in check and keep your body in the fat-burning zone, eat carbs in moderation. They constitute about 30 to 40 percent of my daily calorie intake. Eat enough to keep your glycogen stores loaded, and always eat them in combination with other foods.

### 3. Eat a High-Protein Diet

If you're trying to keep fat off and muscle on, eating protein is second to none. Proteins, like chicken breast and egg whites, build muscle and are the least likely nutrients to be converted to fat and increase fat stores. Protein will also help our fat-loss efforts because, as clinical studies have shown, it causes a greater increase in our metabolisms than any other macronutrient. In other words, the body burns a substantial amount of calories just in the process of breaking down protein. Plus, as I mentioned earlier, protein is also a very potent appetite suppressant. No need for those over-the-counter appetite control pills when we're on a high-protein diet.

Now the big question is, how often and how much protein should we eat each day? Well, it's a fact that muscles grow because of net protein synthesis, which is the difference between protein degradation and synthesis. In the average couch potato, this net difference is zero. He or she isn't causing any muscle damage, so protein requirements are the same day in and day out. If we're bodybuilding or weight training intensely and correctly, we should be causing a good deal of muscle fiber damage, and thus we need extra protein to repair this damage.

As to how much protein we need, some studies show that to elicit muscle growth beyond what we'd normally achieve, we need quite a bit more than the RDA of 70 or so grams. I personally make sure to get *at least* one gram per pound of my lean body weight. For example, if I weigh 200 pounds and have a body fat percentage of 5 percent, my lean body mass is 190 pounds, so I'd make sure to get at least 190 grams of protein, preferably more, each day divided among my six meals.

## 4. Eat Foods in Combination at All Meals

Combining protein, carbs, and fat at every meal slows down the absorption of food, which makes you less likely to gain weight.

Here's why: fats and proteins both lower the *glycemic index* of carbs so we don't get a big fat-producing insulin surge, which leads to weight gain. Fat especially slows down the absorption of anything combined with it. That's why one nice trick is to put a little *all-natural* peanut butter—and I stress only all-natural peanut butter, which lists peanuts or peanuts and salt as the sole ingredients—on our bread or rice cakes and why adding a teaspoon of flaxseed oil to a protein drink or fat-free yogurt is a good idea. This way it takes our bodies a while to absorb these foods and the nutrients are parceled out over time.

As many of you may already have guessed, this technique also allows us to eat some of the higher GI foods without being limited to meal after meal of low GI carbs like oatmeal.

Adding fat to our protein or carbohydrate meals also gives us a greater feeling of fullness in our stomachs, so we feel more satisfied at the end of a meal. Fats and carbs eaten in combination with protein also have another benefit—they are "protein sparing." When eaten in moderation, carbs and fat will be preferentially broken down by the body and used for energy so the body will be free to use the protein sources for more important activities, like muscle growth.

Now, as always, there's a slight exception to the rule of avoiding the big carb-induced insulin surge: that's immediately after a workout. After hitting the weights for an intense hour, our muscle cells are begging to refill their depleted energy, or glycogen, stores with nutrients. So after our workouts we can deliberately elicit that insulin surge by eating a meal of 50 to 80 grams of carbs—mixing both simple or highly processed carbs and lower glycemic carbs along with about 30 to 40 grams of easily absorbed protein, like whey protein. This is where one of those meal replacement drinks often comes in handy. But right after our workouts is really the *only* time we want to have that insulin spike and gorge our muscle cells with goodies.

## 5. Drink Lots of Water

Muscle is made up of more than 70 percent water. A high-protein diet requires more water as do intense workouts since these both are dehydrating activities. Water is also needed to transport vitamins, minerals, supplements, and even foods throughout our bodies. If our water intake is too low, our muscle fullness decreases, and a toxic buildup of ammonia, urea, uric acid, and other bad stuff can start to accumulate in our bodies. That's why, to stay hydrated and pumped throughout the day, we should make it a point to drink about a gallon of water each day with and in between our six meals.

Those are the basic nutritional principles in the Fitness Made Simple program. Following them will help build muscle and burn fat. However, if you are particularly concerned with fat loss, you need to consider one additional factor.

# CALORIES: WHAT YOU NEED TO KNOW

Weight gain and loss are mathematical events. If you consume more calories than you burn off, you will gain fat. If you burn off more calories than you consume, you will lose fat. When trying to increase definition and lose fat, you have to do everything you can to tip this equation in your favor. You want to create a metabolic deficit, and you do that by eating less and/or exercising more. It's as simple as that.

One word of caution: don't cut calories back too far too fast since that can lead to a *loss* of muscle mass. No one wants that. I think weight loss should be gradual. Start by dropping your carbohydrate intake by 30 to 50 grams a day, lowering your saturated fat intake, and moderating your cheating. If you do those three things while bumping up your cardiovascular activity, you'll be amazed at how fast the fat falls away.

There's another rough guideline I like to follow regarding total calories. The plan goes like this: when trying to lose weight or cut up, I consume a daily total calorie intake of my body weight times 10. For example, I weigh between 195 and 200 pounds, so when I'm cutting up or trying to add more definition, I eat around 2,000 calories a day. I find this helps me lose that extra water and fat weight without sacrificing hard-earned muscle tissue. So, to lose fat I follow this formula:

> **Total calories per day = your weight × 10**

To maintain my current physique and, I hope, continue to gain muscle and lose fat steadily, my total calorie intake would be my body weight times 12. In this case, on a maintenance plan, a 200-pound person would eat around 2,400 calories a day. So, to maintain my body I follow this formula:

> **Total calories per day = your weight × 12**

If I'm trying to gain weight—mostly muscle and I'm not concerned with a little fat coming with it—I'd consume my body weight times 15 in calories. In this case, the same 200-pound person would eat around 3,000 calories per day. Thus, to gain weight (mostly lean muscle) I follow this formula:

> **Total calories per day = your weight × 15**

Once again, these are rough estimates or guidelines. Depending on your metabolism and what supplements you're taking, you may have to make adjustments. You could start by raising or lowering your intake by 100 or 200 calories each day and see where that gets you. I make judgments based on the mirror and how my clothes fit, not by the scale. Whatever you do, though, don't make drastic changes that will result in muscle mass loss or unwanted fat gain.

One other word of caution: don't totally eliminate fat from your diet. As I mentioned earlier, fat is essential for healthy skin and hair, and it's involved in the production of hormones that control a variety of biochemical processes in the body. We also need fat to process body fat metabolism. If we make our fat intake too low, our bodies have a self-defense mechanism that causes them to cling on to the last bit of fat for safety. That's why many dieters reach a point where they just can't lose those last few pounds even when they drop calories lower and lower. One trick to avoid this is to keep or add some good fats—like flaxseed oil, natural peanut butter, or avocados—in your plan and keep fat calories around 20 percent of your total daily calorie intake.

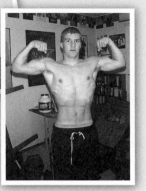

Fitness Made Simple has dramatically increased my fitness level. I was a fat kid growing up, so in my freshman year of high school I started trying to get into shape and trained really hard. The end result was this "before" picture, taken at the end of my senior year.

I then saw a Fitness Made Simple commercial and decided to give it a shot because I still wasn't as cut up as I would have liked to be. It took only my summer vacation to achieve the results of the "after" picture. I give so much praise to FMS that my nickname in college is "Basedow," and I have gotten six other people onto the program.

## WHY IT'S GOOD TO CHEAT

When I'm eating low-calorie and trying to lose fat, I usually have a cheat day—or, as I call it, an *eat day*—every week. On this day I eat whatever I want for a meal or two. This trick helps keep my metabolism high. A low-calorie regimen can drive your metabolism lower and lower over time to compensate for your reduced intake. An eat day here and there helps metabolism stay high by giving your body a bigger influx of nutrients to burn periodically.

We all have unscheduled cheat days when we succumb to cravings. I know I do. When I first started my nutrition plan, I had a lot of them, and I felt terribly guilty. That was wrong. I still have cheat days and I love them. The difference now is that I know I control the cheat days and not the other way around. Before I thought that if I ate a candy bar, I had failed. My nutrition plan was ruined. Now I know that one slip doesn't end my whole program. There will be days when I eat well, and there will be days when I don't. The key is to make the cheat days the *exception* and good eating the rule. I just remember a great bit of advice I once read: "Control is only a moment away. Stop the destructive thing you're doing and you're instantly in control."

As I've said, I don't believe in deprivation. Life is just too short. If I want a brownie, I'll have it. After a few weeks on my nutrition program, however, you won't have the same cravings for cheat foods. Your tastes really do change. It's not that you'll never want cheat foods again, but you won't need them in the same uncontrollable way.

The other benefit of my program is that, since my metabolism is so high now, I can eat my occasional cheat foods—chocolate or whatever—and not even notice a significant difference. Sometimes I'll even have one of my favorite brownies every day for a week and still be able to see great definition in my abs.

It's such a free feeling—it's great. And this is just one small way Fitness Made Simple has changed my life and will change yours.

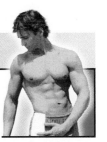

## JOHN-ISM

Fitness is simple. How you look and feel now is the sum total of what you've been doing up to this point. If you don't change what you're doing, you'll keep looking and feeling how you do right now.

# 10 INSIDE TIPS FOR NUTRITION SUCCESS

It's extremely difficult to make a nutrition plan work for you without some inside tips from those who have traveled this road before. So here's what I've learned from my own efforts as well as from the thousands of people who have made my nutrition plan part of their lives:

1. **Write down your food choices and calorie breakdown each day.** This should be done for at least the first couple of weeks, even if you think it's stupid. Believe me, it keeps you more focused and dedicated when you write it down.

2. **Get leftover binge foods out of the house.** The beginning of a new fitness plan is a perfect time for a little pantry cleaning—out with the old and in with the new. Keep only "good" foods in the house. This helps make a habit of eating well, which is especially crucial when changing your food choices during the first few weeks of your program. If you have lots of high-carb and high-fat goodies lying around, get rid of them. Knowing these treats are at arm's reach can make late-night refrigerator raids too tempting. Cheat eating outside of the house stops acting on impulse; it instead allows a moment to think and consciously decide whether it's worth the trip. If I want something and it's worth the trip, I'll get it; if not, I won't.

3. **Shop once a week, every week, for all the food you'll need that week.** Cook at least one day a week, and refrigerate or freeze some meals for later.

4. **If you have a craving, satisfy it and get it over with.** Depriving yourself over and over again will only cause anxiety and depression. It could lead to an even worse binge later. Just try to make better bad choices when you can. If you find yourself at the fast-food drive-through, get the grilled chicken pita instead of the bacon cheeseburger and fries. Taking baby steps like this helps make your nutrition plan easier to follow on a long-term basis.

5. **Try not to eat anything less than two hours before bed.** This practice helps decrease overnight fat storage. Keep carb intake lower during the evening meal and higher during the day, when you're more active and those calories are more likely to be used for energy.

6. **Reward yourself with a nonfood reward.** Treat yourself to a movie or a shopping spree when you accomplish a goal, such as getting through the first week of your nutrition program without cheating. *No accomplishment should go unnoticed or unrewarded.*

7. **Make your goal progress—not perfection.** There are many ways to succeed, but aiming for perfection is the surest way to fail. With your nutrition plan in particular, an obsession with perfection can lead to a preoccupation with food cravings. No one eats perfectly all the time.

8. **If you do cheat or succumb to a craving, don't feel guilty and trash several weeks of good eating for one day of bad.** Your fitness regimen—including your nutrition plan—is a lifelong journey that will have many detours along the way. The truth is that one bad day in most cases will have no lasting visible effect on the gains you have made over several weeks of good days.

9. **Keep in mind that getting through the first couple of weeks of *anything* new is difficult.** You're trying to change a lifetime's worth of habits, and it can't be done in a single day. Trust that you are taking control of your life and changing it for the better. Look to the future with a sense of eagerness and excitement.

10. **And finally, remember that nothing tastes as good as being in great shape feels.**

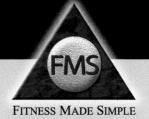

FITNESS MADE SIMPLE

# THE FMS 40

So now you understand the principles of the FMS nutrition plan. You have the key—the right one this time—to unlock the door to the body of your dreams. Follow the rules I laid out, and you'll have more energy and lean muscle than you ever thought possible, all without starving yourself and facing the yo-yo effects of traditional diets.

Rules and principles are great, but I've learned it's crucial to have a specific plan you can follow, particularly when you're first changing the way you eat. As I always say, *failing to plan is the same as planning to fail.*

I don't want you to fail, and that's why I'm going to help you plan. I'm going to explain how you can make sure every meal you eat furthers your efforts to build lean muscle and get rid of fat. I'm going to show you just how varied and delicious a week of eating on the FMS plan can be. I'm even going to give you a few really simple, healthful recipes.

You can't eat right without eating the right foods. If you make fast-food burgers and shakes the centerpiece of your meal plan . . . well, I don't care what else you do—your belly's going to be a whopper and you'll be so large people will call *you* Big Mac.

That's why I've put together the FMS 40—40 super healthful foods that will help you build muscle and get rid of fat. As you'll see, I've divided them by macronutrient into three different groups. There are good-for-you fats that are essential for everything from great hair and great skin to keeping your muscle-developing hormone levels high ("Fantastic Fats"); super sources of protein for building strong, lean muscle ("Muscle-Maximizing Proteins"); and low GI carbs that keep your insulin levels steady and give you all-day energy ("Slow-Burning Carbs").

## JOHN-ISM

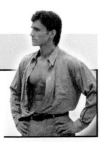

You can make excuses or you can make changes. That choice is always within your power.

# THINK F-M-S

With the FMS 40, planning and making meals is easy. Because I want you to have some of each macronutrient at every meal, you simply choose one or two foods from each column. Just think F-M-S—*Fantastic Fats, Muscle-Maximizing Proteins, Slow-Burning Carbs*—and you're covered.

## The FMS 40

| FANTASTIC FATS | MUSCLE-MAXIMIZING PROTEINS | SLOW-BURNING CARBS |
|---|---|---|
| Flaxseed oil or whole-ground flaxseed meal | Chicken breast | All-natural oatmeal |
| Raw almonds | Turkey breast | Sweet potatoes |
| Raw Brazil nuts | Water-packed tuna | Red potatoes |
| Raw cashews | Wild salmon | Broccoli |
| Raw hazelnuts | Lean red meat | Cauliflower |
| Raw peanuts and other nuts | Egg whites | Spinach |
| Extra-virgin olive oil | Extra-lean ground chicken* | Romaine lettuce |
| Avocados | Extra-lean ground turkey* | String beans |
| All-natural peanut butter | Whey protein powder** | Green and red peppers |
| All-natural almond butter | Low-fat yogurt | Escarole |
| | Tofu** | Apples |
| | Lentils** | Pears |
| | | Bananas |
| | | Berries |
| | | Brown rice |
| | | Hummus |
| | | 100 percent whole-grain breads |
| | | All-natural cereal |

*Read the label closely. Fat and carbs should be close to 0.

**Good protein source for vegetarians

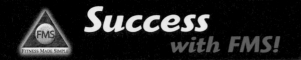
Dear FMS,

I am a father of two, work for a major pharmaceutical company as the director of operations, and with everything that's going on, let's just say I am extremely busy! With this said, I must admit it would be easy to fall into the trap that most people do and make excuses for not exercising/eating well. *John's program has given me the motivation I needed to take the time to improve my physical appearance while improving my health.*

Fitness Made Simple is very easy to follow and has such great nutritional advice. I've told friends and family this is not a diet, certainly not a fad, and it really gives you the tools to make changes to your eating habits without feeling you are being deprived. For

Are the foods on this list the only ones you're allowed to eat on the FMS plan? Of course not. Telling somebody they can't eat a particular food is the surest way I know to make them crave it—and to make them fail when it comes to clean eating. There are lots of other healthful choices out there; plus I know that sometimes you're going to want to indulge in something that's *not* good for you. This is fine occasionally. I never want you to feel deprived.

If you make these 40 foods the foundation of your nutrition plan, however, I believe you'll see amazing changes in the way your body looks, just like I did. You'll also be amazed at how many menu options you have.

most people, it is hard to change your eating patterns without the direction of someone like John. John breaks down what is good to eat, what you should avoid, and when to eat, ultimately giving you the opportunity to see what you otherwise would not have thought possible.

FMS is not a "magic pill" type of plan that sets unrealistic expectations; instead, it's a way of incorporating exercise and nutrition into your life. When I hear people joke, "It's not fair, you look great," I let them know that they, too, can benefit from FMS. I look forward to my continued success and want to give you all at FMS, especially John, a big thank-you.

## JOHN-ISM

Sometimes you win by persistence, by just outlasting the competition.

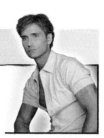

# THE FMS SEVEN-DAY MEAL PLAN

The following is a sample week of eating on the FMS nutrition plan. The daily menus, which use some recipes from this chapter, are guidelines. Feel free to substitute your own healthful choices for variety. Read the labels of all meal ingredients and make serving sizes that fit your caloric needs, as based on your fitness goals.

## MONDAY

**Breakfast**
Egg-white omelet with mixed vegetables

Peanutty Oatmeal Cakes

**Mid-Morning Snack**
1 cup low-fat yogurt with nuts, almonds, or flax meal

**Lunch**
Tuna Pita Delight

**Mid-Afternoon Snack**
Protein bar (any flavor)

Handful of raw almonds or raw mixed nuts

**Dinner**
Light and Tasty Turkey Loaf

Vegetable

Brown rice

Mixed salad with olive oil and vinegar or fat-free, sugar-free balsamic vinaigrette

**Evening Snack**
Protein Shake Fruit Freeze

## TUESDAY

**Breakfast**
All-natural cereal with skim milk

100 percent whole-grain toast with almond butter or peanut butter

**Mid-Morning Snack**
Vanilla protein shake with half an apple or half a banana

**Lunch**
Sliced turkey breast on 100 percent whole-grain bread with a slice of avocado

**Mid-Afternoon Snack**
Hi-Pro Oatmeal Energy Booster

**Dinner**
Chicken Stir-Fry

Romaine lettuce salad with olive oil and vinegar

**Evening Snack**
Protein Shake Fruit Freeze

## WEDNESDAY

**Breakfast**

All-natural oatmeal topped with flax meal

Egg-white omelet with spinach and cut-up chicken breast cubes

**Mid-Morning Snack**

1 cup low-fat yogurt with nuts or almonds

**Lunch**

Extra-lean turkey burger on a 100 percent whole-grain bun or wrapped in lettuce

**Mid-Afternoon Snack**

Protein bar (any flavor)

Handful of raw almonds or raw mixed nuts

**Dinner**

Wild salmon

Vegetable

Spinach salad with olive oil and vinegar

**Evening Snack**

Protein Shake Fruit Freeze

## THURSDAY

**Breakfast**

Egg-white omelet with mixed vegetables

Peanutty Oatmeal Cakes

**Mid-Morning Snack**

Vanilla protein shake with half a banana or half an apple

**Lunch**

Chunky Chicken Salad

**Mid-Afternoon Snack**

Hi-Pro Oatmeal Energy Booster

**Dinner**

Lean red meat

Vegetable

Red potato

Romaine lettuce salad with olive oil and vinegar

**Evening Snack**

Protein Shake Fruit Freeze

## FRIDAY

**Breakfast**
All-natural cereal with skim milk or all-natural oatmeal

100 percent whole-grain toast with all-natural almond butter or all-natural peanut butter

**Mid-Morning Snack**
1 cup low-fat yogurt with raw mixed nuts or raw almonds

**Lunch**
Chicken breast on 100 percent whole-grain bread

**Mid-Afternoon Snack**
Protein bar (any flavor)

Handful of raw almonds or raw mixed nuts

**Dinner**
Mexican Scrambled Omelet

Spinach salad with avocado

**Evening Snack**
Protein Shake Fruit Freeze

## SATURDAY

**Breakfast**
Hi-Pro Oatmeal Energy Booster with flax meal

**Mid-Morning Snack**
1 cup low-fat cottage cheese with fruit and raw mixed nuts (all-natural raw trail mix)

**Lunch**
Tuna Pita Delight

**Mid-Afternoon Snack**
Protein bar (any flavor)

**Dinner**
Turkey or chicken breast

Brown rice

Vegetable

Romaine lettuce salad with olive oil and vinegar

**Evening Snack**
Protein Shake Fruit Freeze

## SUNDAY

**Eat Day!** Follow the regular schedule from your other "good eating" days, but indulge with something you've been craving. Don't go crazy, watch overall calories, but enjoy yourself.

## THE **REVERSE** MEAL TRIANGLE

In my mind America is the greatest country in the world, but there's no denying that we're also the fattest. In part that's because many of us have things ass-backward when it comes to our meals. Too many people in this country eat little or no breakfast, have a big lunch, and then devour an even more enormous dinner. All of that is the complete opposite of our caloric needs throughout the day, and it leads to unnecessary binging and unhealthy fat storage.

Instead, I like to follow an approach I call the Reverse Meal Triangle, with the biggest meal of the day, breakfast, at the top and the smallest meal of the day, dinner, at the bottom. As I like to put it, you should:

- Eat breakfast like a king.
- Eat lunch like a prince.
- Eat dinner like a pauper.

Eating a large breakfast and a moderate lunch gives you the calories you need for energy throughout the day. By eating a smaller dinner, you avoid a big evening caloric surge that can lead to unwanted fat storage, particularly in trouble-prone areas like the love handles in men and the waist, hips, and thighs in women.

# FMS RECIPES

Here are a few of the best fat-fighting and muscle-building recipes I've tried and thousands of other FMS members are using to build lean, defined physiques. I hope they'll help you accomplish all of your fitness goals as well. You'll see some of these recipes included in the FMS sample meal plan. For variety, you can substitute others as long as you keep the macronutrient breakdowns and total calories consistent.

## HOW MUCH SHOULD YOU EAT?

Yes, size does matter. When I first started out, I used to drive myself crazy by weighing and measuring foods, but I learned to make things simpler. I now go by portion sizes. A portion is roughly the size of my clenched fist or the palm of my hand. When I'm trying to increase definition or get leaner, I make sure my protein and complex carb portions for each meal are that size. If I'm eating out, which I love to do, I simply bring home any extra food to enjoy later.

Don't feel that you have to finish what's on your plate. If you are like me and had it ingrained that you must consume everything placed in front of you because there are people starving in Ethiopia, try using smaller plates. Switching to smaller china or, in my case, paper plates is a way to feel that sense of accomplishment you get from cleaning your plate—without overeating.

# *Mexican Scrambled Omelet*

**YOU'LL NEED**  4 ounces extra-lean ground turkey breast

5 egg whites

¼ cup salsa or picante sauce

1 cup mixed red and green peppers and mushrooms

½ cup cooked brown rice

½ teaspoon chili powder

**DIRECTIONS**  Use a nonstick frying pan or spray zero-calorie nonstick spray on a regular frying pan. Divide ground turkey breast into little balls or bits. Add egg whites, salsa, vegetables, rice, and chili powder with turkey in the pan. Heat on medium setting on the stove, and mix periodically with a wooden spoon until eggs begin to brown and turkey is cooked (pink color disappears). Sometimes it's a good idea to cook the turkey bits beforehand, but it's usually not necessary. Remove from stove and put on a plate.

*Makes 1 serving and takes less than 5 minutes to prepare (time estimate is based on using precooked brown rice)*

320 calories (50g protein, 25g carbs, 2g fat)

# *Super Protein Pancakes*

**YOU'LL NEED**     ³/₄ cup 100 percent whole-grain flour

1 teaspoon baking powder

¹/₄ teaspoon salt (optional)

1 packet zero-calorie artificial sweetener

1 24-gram scoop unflavored whey protein powder

¹/₂ cup skim milk

2 egg whites

Zero-calorie nonstick cooking spray

**DIRECTIONS**     Place flour, baking powder, salt, sweetener, and protein powder in a large bowl. Mix by hand. Add milk and egg whites in that order, mixing by hand after each addition. Set the mixture aside.

Drop by scant ¹/₄ cups onto a nonstick skillet coated with cooking spray, heated to medium-low. Once pancakes have bubbles that are beginning to pop, flip and cook until just browned on the other side.

*Makes 2 servings and takes less than 10 minutes to prepare*

100 percent whole-grain flour: 230 calories (22g protein, 37g carbs, 1g fat)

# *Peanutty Oatmeal Cakes*

**YOU'LL NEED**  1/2 tablespoon all-natural peanut butter (must list only *peanuts* or *peanuts and salt* as ingredients)

2 rice cakes

1 packet zero-calorie artificial sweetener

1/2 teaspoon cinnamon

1/2 cup cooked all-natural oatmeal

**DIRECTIONS**  Spread all-natural peanut butter on rice cakes. Mix artificial sweetener and cinnamon into cooked plain oatmeal. Spread oatmeal on top of peanut butter on rice cakes. Eat and enjoy.

*Makes 1 serving and takes less than 5 minutes to prepare (oatmeal cooking time is 1 1/2 minutes)*

165 calories (7g protein, 18g carbs, 7g fat)

# *Chunky Chicken Salad*

**YOU'LL NEED**   Salad consisting of romaine lettuce, tomatoes, red and green peppers, mushrooms, carrots, and any other favorite vegetable

4 ounces grilled chicken breast

1 tablespoon flaxseed oil, olive oil, or oil and vinegar dressing

**DIRECTIONS**   Toss salad and mix in chicken breast. Add dressing and serve.

*Makes 1 serving and takes less than 5 minutes to prepare*

310 calories (26g protein, 20g carbs, 14g fat)

# Shrimp Salad

**YOU'LL NEED**   1 medium carrot, diced fine

2 ribs of celery, diced fine

½ pound peeled medium shrimp, cooked

Juice of 1 lemon

Boston or romaine lettuce leaves

1 tablespoon low-calorie cocktail sauce

**DIRECTIONS**   Place carrot and celery in a medium bowl. Cut each shrimp into three pieces. Place in the bowl. Add lemon juice and mix. Serve atop a few lettuce leaves. Use cocktail sauce sparingly for dipping.

*Makes 2 servings and takes less than 10 minutes to prepare*

140 calories (25g protein, 8g carbs, 1.5g fat)

## ENTRÉES

# Ground Beef, Bean, and Corn Burritos

**YOU'LL NEED**

*For the beef (can substitute extra-lean ground turkey)*

½ pound 93 percent lean ground beef

1 teaspoon ground cumin seed

¼ teaspoon garlic powder

¼ teaspoon onion powder

⅛ teaspoon dried Mexican oregano leaves

½ teaspoon low-calorie or calorie-free seasoning (e.g., Mrs. Dash)

⅛ teaspoon ground black pepper

Pinch cayenne pepper

*For the beans*

1 15-ounce can black beans, drained but not rinsed

1¼ teaspoons ground cumin seed

¼ teaspoon garlic powder

½ teaspoon onion powder

⅛ teaspoon dried Mexican oregano leaves

½ teaspoon low-calorie or calorie-free seasoning (e.g., Mrs. Dash)

¼ teaspoon ground black pepper

Pinch cayenne pepper

1 tablespoon low-sodium mild salsa

½ 10-ounce package frozen corn, thawed

4 100 percent whole-grain tortillas

¼ cup reduced-fat shredded sharp cheddar or reduced-fat Mexican blend cheese (optional)

¼ medium avocado, chopped

**DIRECTIONS** *To prepare the beef:* Preheat a heavy skillet on medium heat. Place beef in the skillet. Add spices and cook, stirring frequently, until beef is fully browned. Set aside.

*To prepare the beans:* Place beans in a medium saucepan over low heat. Add spices and salsa. Cook covered for 15 to 20 minutes.

*To prepare the corn:* Follow package directions.

*To assemble burritos:* Warm tortillas, covered by a wet paper towel, in the microwave on high for 30 seconds. Place about ¼ cup each of beans, meat, and corn in a stripe down the center of the tortilla. Top with cheese (optional) and avocado. Wrap and serve immediately.

*Makes 2 servings and takes less than 20 minutes to prepare*

Ground beef without cheese: 570 calories (42g protein, 92g carbs, 11g fat)
Ground beef with cheese: 620 calories (46g protein, 92g carbs, 14g fat)
Ground turkey without cheese: 560 calories (48g protein, 92g carbs, 8g fat)
Ground turkey with cheese: 610 calories (52g protein, 92g carbs, 11g fat)

# Beef Tenderloin in Balsamic Reduction

**YOU'LL NEED**    ¼ teaspoon low-calorie or calorie-free seasoning (e.g., Mrs. Dash)

½ pound beef tenderloin, cut to 1- to 1½-inch thickness
(use USDA Choice)

1 tablespoon extra-virgin olive oil

⅓ cup balsamic vinegar

**DIRECTIONS**    Bring a heavy skillet (cast iron is best) up to medium or medium-high heat. While the pan is preheating, rub the seasoning into the meat thoroughly on both sides, using more or less depending on your particular taste. Pour oil into the pan. Place tenderloin into the pan. Cover with a splatter guard. Cook until the meat is brown one-third of the way up the side of the cut. Turn and cook until desired doneness is reached. Use an instant-read meat thermometer to measure doneness. Tenderloin is best served rare to medium. Remove steaks to a serving platter. Turn the heat up to medium high, and pour 2 tablespoons of water in the skillet. Immediately follow with balsamic vinegar. Stir the mixture around, thoroughly working in all the pan drippings. Once the mixture has reduced its volume by half, pour it over the meat. Serve.

*Makes 2 servings and takes less than 15 minutes to prepare*

210 calories (22g protein, 5g carbs, 11g fat)

# *Turkey Meatballs*

**YOU'LL NEED**   ½ pound extra-lean ground turkey breast (fat content should be less than 3 grams per serving)

¼ cup rolled oats

1½ tablespoons tomato ketchup

½ teaspoon low-calorie or calorie-free seasoning (e.g., Mrs. Dash)

½ tablespoon olive oil

½ small onion, minced

**DIRECTIONS**   Place turkey in a medium bowl. Add oats, ketchup, and seasoning. Mix by hand and form into meatballs 1 inch in diameter. Set aside. Place olive oil in a heavy-bottomed skillet on medium heat. When oil is hot, sauté onion until translucent. Add meatballs, being sure not to crowd the pan. Cook until brown on all sides and the interior of a tested meatball shows no pink. You may be required to prepare two or more batches to cook all the turkey. Serve with your choice of low-calorie, low-fat sauce for dipping.

*Makes 2 servings and takes less than 20 minutes to prepare*

210 calories (30g protein, 13g carbs, 6g fat)

# Light and Tasty Turkey Loaf

**YOU'LL NEED**  1 packet meatloaf mix (e.g., Adolph's, which consists of both a sauce and a bread crumb mix; omit the bread crumb portion if you are monitoring carb calories)

1½ cups plus ½ cup cold water

2 pounds (32 ounces) extra-lean ground turkey breast

4 egg whites

2 teaspoons low-calorie or calorie-free spicy seasoning (e.g., Mrs. Dash)

**DIRECTIONS**  Preheat oven to 350°F. Combine sauce portion of meatloaf mix with ½ cup cold water until it reaches a thick, pasty consistency. Then add 1½ cups water and mix thoroughly. In a large bowl combine meat, egg whites, bread crumb portion of meatloaf mix (optional), and 1 cup of the sauce mixture. Mix thoroughly, making sure there are no clumps of bread crumbs. Then add up to 2 teaspoons seasoning if you like your meatloaf spicy. Mix thoroughly again. Shape the mixture in a baking tray and place in the oven for about 60 minutes. You can also spray a baking tray or meatloaf pan with zero-calorie nonstick vegetable oil or olive oil cooking spray to avoid sticking. After about 60 minutes, take the turkey loaf out of the oven and spread the remaining sauce over the top and sides. Place in the oven for an additional 10 to 15 minutes or until cooked fully. Take out of the oven and serve. Refrigerate individual servings in foil or plastic containers to eat later in the week.

*Makes 8 servings and takes 90 minutes to prepare*

160 calories (29g protein, 7g carbs, 1.5g fat)

# *Chicken Stir-Fry*

**YOU'LL NEED**   $1/2$ tablespoon extra-virgin olive oil

2 cups mixed vegetables: mushrooms, peapods, red and green peppers, water chestnuts, carrots, onions, broccoli, cauliflower, etc.

4 ounces grilled chicken breast (can substitute turkey breast)

1 teaspoon low-sodium teriyaki or soy sauce (optional)

**DIRECTIONS**   Add olive oil to a frying pan and then add mixed vegetables, chicken breast, and teriyaki or soy sauce. Heat on medium setting for 2 to 3 minutes, making sure to mix with a wooden spoon.

*Makes 1 serving and takes less than 5 minutes to prepare*

220 calories (26g protein, 11g carbs, 8g fat)

# *Tuna Pita Delight*

**YOU'LL NEED**   ½ 6-ounce can water-packed, low-sodium, chunk light or white tuna

¼ to ½ cup diced vegetables: lettuce, tomato, cauliflower, and bean sprouts (feel free to add some of your other favorites as well)

½ tablespoon olive oil

½ tablespoon balsamic vinegar

1 fat-free pita

**DIRECTIONS**   Rinse and drain tuna at least three times. In a bowl

combine vegetables, olive oil, balsamic vinegar, and tuna.

Mix thoroughly and put inside pita.

*Makes 1 serving and takes less than 5 minutes to prepare*

345 calories (27g protein, 41g carbs, 8g fat)

# *Protein Shake Fruit Freeze*

**YOU'LL NEED**   2 24-gram scoops of whey protein powder

1 packet zero-calorie artificial sweetener

½ tablespoon flaxseed oil

½ cup frozen fruit (best choices: strawberries, blueberries, bananas, cherries)

7 to 12 ice cubes

**DIRECTIONS**   In a blender combine protein powder, artificial sweetener, flaxseed oil, and frozen fruit with ice cubes. Blend on "grate" speed for about a minute to bring the mixture to a foamy thickness. The more ice cubes you add, the thicker the shake becomes. It often tastes best when it reaches a slushy consistency and can be eaten with a spoon if you want.

*Makes 1 serving and takes about 3 minutes to prepare (a great after-workout, high-protein drink)*

225 calories (26g protein, 12g carbs, 9g fat)

# Jell-O Fruit Jubilee

**YOU'LL NEED**

2 cups boiling water

2 0.6-ounce boxes sugar-free Jell-O (your favorite flavor)

2 cups cold water

½ cup apple slices

½ cup pear slices

½ cup mixed berries: blueberries, strawberries, raspberries, etc.

**DIRECTIONS**

In a large bowl or plastic container add boiling water to the two boxes of sugar-free Jell-O. Stir with a fork until all the powder is dissolved, usually about 2 minutes. Add cold water and stir again. Add apples, pears, and berries. Cover the container with a lid or cling wrap and refrigerate overnight until the mixture gels. If you want the fruit to be in suspension in the Jell-O, put the Jell-O in the refrigerator for about 2 hours before adding the fruit so it can reach a thicker consistency.

*Makes 8 servings and takes less than 5 minutes to prepare (plus refrigeration time)*

20 calories (1g protein, 4g carbs, 0g fat)

# *Choco-Peanut Clusters*

**YOU'LL NEED**   1 1.4-ounce box Jell-O fat-free, sugar-free instant chocolate pudding mix

2 cups cold water

1 tablespoon all-natural crunchy peanut butter

2 rice cakes broken into fourths

**DIRECTIONS**   Prepare pudding with water, according to directions on the box. Spread peanut butter on rice cakes. Heat rice cakes in the microwave for 30 seconds (optional). Dip rice cakes with peanut butter into one serving (i.e., one-fourth) of cold chocolate pudding. Eat and enjoy. Remaining pudding can be refrigerated.

*Makes 1 serving and takes less than 5 minutes to prepare*

265 calories (10g protein, 41g carbs, 7g fat)

# Hi-Pro Oatmeal Energy Booster

**YOU'LL NEED**

$\frac{1}{2}$ cup uncooked all-natural oatmeal

2 24-gram scoops of whey protein powder

$\frac{1}{4}$ cup diced apples or pears

1 packet zero-calorie artificial sweetener

$\frac{1}{2}$ teaspoon cinnamon

$\frac{1}{2}$–1 cup water

**DIRECTIONS**

Combine oatmeal with protein powder, diced fruit, artificial sweetener, and cinnamon. Add water to get the desired consistency. Mix together and heat in the microwave for $1\frac{1}{2}$ minutes. You can vary fruit choices to your taste.

*Makes 1 serving and takes less than 5 minutes to prepare*

285 calories (30g protein, 30g carbs, 5g fat)

# John's FMS Personal Pizza

**YOU'LL NEED**   3 ounces extra-lean ground turkey breast

1 cup of mixed diced mushrooms, red and green peppers, onions, tomatoes, and spinach

1 fat-free whole-grain pita

Fat-free shredded cheese (a couple of pinches)

**DIRECTIONS**   Use a nonstick frying pan or spray zero-calorie nonstick spray on a regular frying pan. Break up the turkey breast into small bits and put them, along with the diced vegetables, into the frying pan. Heat on medium setting on the stove, mixing occasionally with a wooden spoon or spatula until the turkey breast becomes slightly brown. Put the turkey breast and vegetables on the pita, sprinkle the fat-free shredded cheese on top, and then place in the microwave for about a minute, just enough time for the cheese to begin to melt.

**Note:** If I'm in the mood for a Mexican pizza, I'll add black bean salsa as a sauce. For an Italian pizza, low-fat or fat-free tomato sauce is great. And for a vegetarian pizza, diced mixed vegetables with tofu does the trick.

*Makes 1 serving and takes less than 5 minutes to prepare*

250 calories (31g protein, 29g carbs, ½g fat)

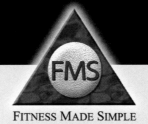

FITNESS MADE SIMPLE

# CHAPTER 6

# THE FIRST FOUR WEEKS

I'm not going to lie to you. Trying to change the way you eat might not be easy at first. It certainly wasn't simple for me back when I gave up my fast-food-burger and chocolate-brownie-cake routine. I've never done drugs, but I imagine that getting over the sugar cravings I had was almost like an addict kicking a habit. It was miserable.

Why? It's certainly not because our bodies need bad stuff to live on. Believe me, no one was born to crave sugar or saturated fat. I didn't come out of the womb needing a brownie and a 10-pack of White Castles at midnight. I wanted them because that was what I had been eating for

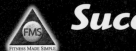
John,

FMS changed my life. I have to admit that it was really your physique that made the initial impact. I've been working out for years but never before achieved such a ripped state. Witnessing your absolutely shredded condition provided all the motivation I needed! The FMS program then provided the tools.

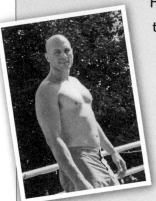

After a few weeks of monitoring my nutritional intake and watching my carbs very closely, something happened. My body began to burn the fuel more efficiently. I was getting hungry every few hours and I could almost feel my skin getting tighter. This was all the additional support I needed to complete a couple months of perfect nutrition and brief but focused workouts. You see the results.

I'm all about living an extraordinary life. FMS has helped to give me the vehicle I need to actively and energetically pursue that life.

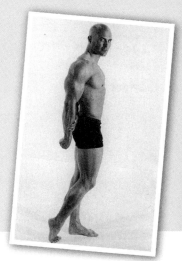

a long time. Your body doesn't give a damn about how you look; your body just wants to survive. So if it's been living on what you've been feeding it more than X number of years, that's what it's going to crave.

It's another one of those dirty tricks nature plays on us. Your mind may want to turn on a dime—*I want to look better, I want to feel better*—but your body is about four or so weeks behind your mind. It takes that long to stop craving the crap and start craving new, better foods.

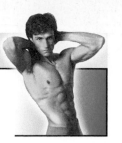

## JOHN-ISM
You can always be better;
FMS shows you how.

But it will happen.

After that first month or so, I no longer woke up in the middle of the night with images of brownies dancing around my head, and I was no longer compelled to stop at every single White Castle I passed by. I didn't feel like I was depriving myself, either. I had simply gotten past a biological reality over which I had no control.

The same thing will happen to you. After about four weeks, you're not going to want junk anymore. When you do take a bite of it, you're going to think, *Do I even want a second bite?* That's the way I feel about chocolate. I have a little piece of chocolate every day. Before it would take three-quarters of a chocolate brownie cake to satisfy me. Now one little square of a dark chocolate bar is more than enough.

## THE POWER OF WRITING IT DOWN

How can you make it through those first four weeks? When I first started following the FMS nutrition plan, one of the most powerful tools I had was a little notebook that I carried with me everywhere. In it I wrote every single thing I ate, broken down into calories, along with grams of protein, carbs, and fat.

For the first month that you're following the plan, I recommend you do the same. To make things easy you can photocopy the food journal here or buy your own little notebook. It's crucial not only for learning the

Dear Fitness Made Simple,

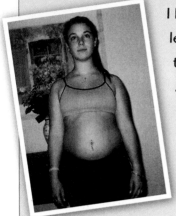

I have never regularly worked out so much in my life! My energy levels have definitely risen and I feel so much better. It's so hard to get myself to exercise, but when I do I just feel great afterward. All my old excuses about how I didn't have enough time to work out or I had something else to do seem like so much hot air now.

I want to thank Fitness Made Simple for improving my health and lifestyle!

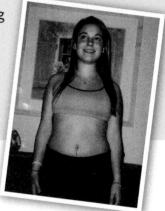

nutritional breakdown of foods but even more for the mental side of changing your nutrition habits. If you're tempted to eat something that's not part of the FMS plan, the fact that you have to write it down may stop you from giving in to the impulse. You know it's going to be indelibly written in your journal and, boy, are you going to feel like an ass at night if you see that you overate needlessly during the day. Keeping a food journal gives you control, and control is what the FMS plan is all about.

## JOHN-ISM

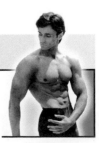

The true mark of a star is being able to shine through difficult times.

# FMS FOOD JOURNAL

| FOOD | CALORIES | CARBS | PROTEIN | FAT |
|---|---|---|---|---|
| | | | | |
| | | | | |
| | | | | |
| | | | | |
| | | | | |
| | | | | |
| | | | | |
| | | | | |
| | | | | |
| | | | | |
| | | | | |
| | | | | |
| | | | | |

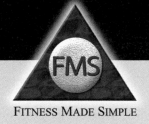

FITNESS MADE SIMPLE

# NUTRITION
## FAQS

Even though the FMS nutrition plan is simple to follow, people occasionally have questions about the program's finer points or what they should do in certain specific situations. Here are some of the questions I'm most commonly asked about the FMS nutrition plan and my recommendations for what to do.

# CONQUER CRAVINGS

*What's the best way to handle food cravings during the day?*

I have three little "tricks" that I use regularly to keep cheating urges at bay.

1. Have lots of crunchy vegetables, like broccoli, cauliflower, and carrots, around whenever you get that cheating feeling. Bulky, fibrous veggies are unbelievably filling and nutrient-dense, but they're exceedingly low in calories.

2. Keep sugar-free Jell-O on hand to avoid late-night binges. Jell-O is tasty, fun to eat, and almost devoid of calories. Splurging on the entire box adds only a minor 40 calories to your daily plan.

3. My third trick involves sugar-free gum. Sometimes on long car rides or during very stressful days you just get the urge to chew something, even when you're not necessarily hungry. At this time a stick of gum works wonders to get your mind off cheating.

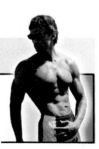

## JOHN-ISM

If you can't envision yourself with a great body living a great life, you'll probably never get there, but if you keep that image in your head every day and dedicate yourself to achieving it, you just might be surprised by how quickly it turns into reality.

# ENOUGH IS ENOUGH

*How can I make sure I don't overeat at mealtime?*

As I mentioned in my Top 10 Tips for Living Lean and Healthy, your goal should be to leave the table when you're no longer hungry, not when you're full. This can be tough, however, because of the 15- to 20-minute lag time between when your stomach has had enough and your brain sends the message that you should stop eating.

This is why I encourage people to brush their teeth or have a piece of sugar-free gum when they want to end a meal. Both make additional food distasteful, and they signal to your body that the meal is over. Doing this can help you avoid overeating and keep unwanted pounds off your trouble-prone areas.

# DINING OUT

*The FMS plan sounds great when I'm eating at home, but what if I go to a restaurant?*

You don't have to be a shut-in. I wasn't, and I don't ever want to hear the excuse that it's too hard to eat out. Instead, you just need to follow four simple rules when you're at a restaurant.

1. **Order something healthful, even if it's not on the menu.** Just about every restaurant now offers healthful alternatives, so finding something good to eat shouldn't be that difficult. If you can't, however, don't let that stop you. Order something healthful whether you see it on the menu or not. Don't just accept the food as is. If you go to an Italian restaurant because that's where your friends

John,

I have all six of your DVDs and I'm very serious about getting into shape. I have worked out with weights faithfully three times a week since receiving your tapes and I'm really watching what I eat.

I am 44 years old and have never felt better. I've gone from 30 percent body fat to 25 percent so far, and I have dropped from a size 9 pants to a size 5. I still need a lot of work on my lower abs, but I'm seeing a big difference. Three C-sections and a lower back problem don't help matters, but I have seen a tremendous improvement in my back. It's getting much stronger and flares up only a fraction of what it used to. Thanks!

---

want to eat, ask for a plain chicken breast on a salad and remember that you can make special requests, like sauce on the side, steamed instead of fried, or cooked without oil. Don't feel timid about it. Keep in mind that the meal you're eating out would probably cost about one-fifth the price if you made it at home. You're paying for the service; it's OK to make them work for it.

For example, when I'm going out to breakfast, I commonly request egg-white omelets cooked with calorie-free nonstick spray and no cheese. If I watch out for the hidden sources of fat and calories that I don't even enjoy, I'm then able to incorporate some very palatable cheat foods, such as a small piece of dark chocolate cake, into my meal plan every once in a while without noticing any negative effects on my muscle definition or body fat level.

In phone consultations I often tell people who've ordered my Fitness Made Simple videos, "It's not the little piece of cake that makes you fat—it's all your other daily sources of excess carbs and fat combined with the cake that makes you fat."

2. **Get a doggie bag.** Some restaurants these days serve portion sizes that could feed a small country. You don't have to finish everything on your plate. Even when I go to big important business meetings, I always take home a doggie bag. This serves two purposes: number 1, you're sticking to your nutrition plan because you're controlling portion sizes; number 2, it brings back all the wonderful memories of the restaurant when you have it later that day or the next day.

3. **Watch the bread and chips prior to your meal.** Most people don't mentally count these as part of the meal. They may be cost-free, but they're sure not calorie-free.

4. **Don't worry about being considered a pain or picky by your friends or the restaurant staff when you're making a special order.** Once again, remember you're paying for this service, and, as for your friends, after they see the results of your efforts, they'll probably start following your lead.

## JOHN-ISM

Believe in yourself and you can accomplish anything!

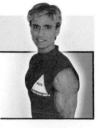

# THINK BEFORE YOU DRINK

*Am I allowed to drink alcohol when I'm following the FMS plan?*

No food or drink is outlawed in the FMS nutrition plan. Doing so would just make you want it more. The key is to practice moderation. When it comes to calories, beer, wine, and alcohol are no worse, and probably better, than chocolate or pizza. They're simple carbs, but they're manageable if you don't overdo them. If you make clean eating the rule and cheating the exception, one little indulgence here and there isn't going to have a noticeable impact on the physique you're trying to build.

If you're used to having a beer every single night and you find this habit is holding you back, take a baby step forward—have a beer every other night or have half the serving size and see if that improves your fitness results. You always want to make better choices, but you don't want to deprive yourself. Remember, your fitness program shouldn't be something that makes you miserable. It should be a lifestyle change to make you both physically and mentally better.

# PARTY PLANNING

*Parties, particularly around the holidays, are my downfall. How do I avoid blowing my diet during the party season?*

First of all, you're not going on a diet—you're adopting a new fitness lifestyle and giving yourself a nutrition plan. Second, having a few too many goodies at a holiday party doesn't mean you've blown it. In most cases, as I've stated many times, one bad day of eating will have little impact on your overall efforts to get lean.

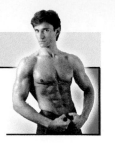

## JOHN-ISM

Change your mind, change
your world.

That said, there are some strategies I use to give myself more control when I know I'm going to a party. The most important thing is
to never arrive at a party hungry. Have a small meal or snack that's
part of your nutrition plan an hour or so before you go out. I also like
to drink plenty of water beforehand, at least 8 to 16 ounces, which
helps fill up my stomach. You'll still be able to enjoy some of your
cheat foods, but you're not going to have a ravenous binge at the party
because you really won't want to.

## SWEET TOOTH

*I love dessert. How can I indulge my sweet tooth while still sticking to
the FMS plan?*

If you can, go without dessert. If you can't, however, you want to try to
make better bad choices. There are a lot of sugar-free, fat-free alternatives out there, which are a step in the right direction and also taste
great. Sugar-free dark chocolate, for instance, is just amazing. If you're
craving something particularly decadent and it's your cheat day, share
it with a friend or two and just eat a third of the portion. Once again,
the idea is to gain control. The best part is, after a few weeks of eating
cleanly, you're not going to want to have a massive amount of dessert.

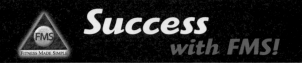
Hi John,

I love the straightforward and easy-to-follow FMS nutrition and training plan. It's a program that finally makes my goals seem attainable!

Thanks again for your guidance. I just wanted to update you on my progress. I am now on week #6 with a weight of 166 pounds and 12 percent body fat. I feel good and hard and seem to be maintaining my muscle well. I also seem to be getting a better handle on my carb intake. Here is my progress so far:

**WEEK 1:** 177 pounds and 17 percent body fat
**WEEK 4:** 169 pounds and 14 percent body fat
**WEEK 6:** 166 pounds and 12 percent body fat

I have been training for about 12 years now. Your program is the best out there, and, believe me, I have tried them all.

## PROTEIN POWER

*I'm a vegetarian. How can I make sure I get enough protein?*

Getting 30 to 40 percent of your calories from protein is more of a challenge for vegetarians, but it can be done. In addition to lentils, tofu, and low-fat, nongelatin-based yogurt, all of which are good protein sources, I also recommend whey protein shakes and egg-white omelets. I almost treat my omelets like soup, throwing in whatever extra vegetables I happen to have handy. This variety keeps me from getting bored while enjoying the protein-packed benefits of the omelet.

# PACKING ON POUNDS

*Unlike a lot of people, I've always felt too skinny and I actually want to gain weight. How can I adjust the FMS plan so that I pack on a few pounds of lean muscle?*

Three words: eat more calories. Just make sure they're quality calories. Here are the formulas I follow: If I'm trying to lose fat, I eat my body weight times 10 in calories each day. If I'm trying to maintain my weight, I eat my body weight times 12. If I'm trying to gain muscle and I'm not concerned with a little fat gain, I eat my body weight times 15. Everything else about the FMS nutrition plan, including the macronutrient breakdowns for each meal, stays the same.

# AN APPLE A DAY?

*People always say that fruit is a healthful snack. Do you recommend eating a lot of it?*

A little fruit each day is good, but not too much. If you're trying to get lean, fruits are tricky since they contain fructose (sugar), which is easily converted into body fat. I like to stick with the harder and more fibrous fruits, such as apples and pears, along with bananas, which are high in potassium, to put in my protein shakes. Fruit is your friend, but keep it in moderation.

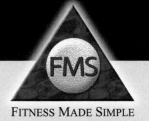

FITNESS MADE SIMPLE

# EXERCISE
## MADE
## SIMPLE

Now that you have a nutrition plan in place, it's time to get to work making your muscles grow.

A lot of people think having a lean, muscular body is like winning the lottery, something that happens only by chance. They look at the muscle definition I have and say, "Oh, you must be genetically gifted." That's BS. Nobody in my family has visible abs. Sure, good genes probably help some people, but I got the body of my dreams by understanding physiology and then developing a training program that works with nature, not against it. By following the FMS plan, you can do the same thing.

## JOHN-ISM

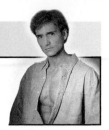

Don't ever settle for less than what you want. It sets a bad precedent. Once you settle for less than what makes you happy in one area of your life, it spreads like a cancer throughout every other aspect. Settle-itis, as I call it, is a nasty disease that ruins lives. Never settle; always strive to be better.

As with my nutrition plan, I went through a lot of trial and error—with an emphasis on error—when it came to finding an exercise plan that would really develop my muscles. I tried all-cardio programs and no-cardio programs. I tried lifting "heavy" one day a week. I tried spending multiple hours in the gym every single day. I made some gains, I guess, but none of the training programs gave me the lean, hard body I was looking for. I was frustrated, didn't really like working out anymore, and had reached a point where I could have thrown up my hands and said, "Oh, this is the body God gave me—may as well just accept it."

I could have come down with a pretty nasty case of "settle-itis."

But I didn't. Instead, I figured out two things that have become the cornerstones of my exercise philosophy. First, *fitness is not a game of how miserable you can make yourself. You have to find a routine you enjoy—not one that you can tolerate, but one that you actually enjoy and look forward to.* If you don't, it will never become part of your lifestyle, and making exercise part of your day is the key not only to changing your body but also to changing your life. The FMS plan is one I can't wait to do every day.

My other exercise key is this: *more is not always better.* You don't have to spend countless hours in the gym every day to get the body you want. The goal is to train smarter, not harder.

The FMS workout program has three components: cardiovascular exercise, strength training with weights, and ab training. In the following sections I'll show you how to approach each one and work all three into your life.

And again, you don't have to join a gym to do my program. Some folks like the gym (I'm one of them), but the entire FMS plan can be done at home with a simple set of adjustable dumbbells and a bench. That's all you need to craft a lean, strong, muscular form. Many of the greatest FMS successes have come from people who exercised at home.

But if, like me, you prefer working out in the gym, select one that you find to be comfortable and that is not too far from your house. Nothing kills a workout faster than a long commute. Convenience is key when incorporating fitness into your life and sticking with your program over time. You need to be sure that whatever gym you select is well equipped, but don't get too hung up on the latest machines. The vibe and location are much more important. Plus I still believe basic free weights—dumbbells and barbells—help sculpt bodies better than most of the newfangled stuff.

## CARDIO: FOUR OR FIVE DAYS PER WEEK, FIRST THING IN THE MORNING

When it comes to cardio, timing is everything. I think it's best to do it four or five days a week, first thing in the morning before breakfast, especially when your primary goal is to lose fat. One study I saw says you burn 200 percent more fat if you do cardio right after you wake up on an empty

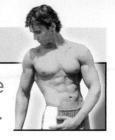

stomach. At that point your blood-sugar and insulin levels are low and stable, and your body is more inclined to burn stored fat for energy. In fact, morning cardio is your fat cells' worst nightmare.

Any low-impact exercise is fine—elliptical trainer, stationary bike, treadmill, walking, and even dancing. The important thing is that you enjoy doing it. Aim for an intensity that lets you carry on a conversation without losing your breath; in other words, you should be able to talk in full sentences while working out. If you're huffing and puffing, you could be working too hard and breaking down muscle tissue. Work your way up to 40 to 50 minutes per session. If you can do only 10 or 15 minutes when you start out, that's fine. Just try to do a little bit more each time. Remember: baby steps.

If for some reason you can't do your cardio first thing in the morning, the second-best time is immediately after your strength workout. Your insulin and blood-sugar levels are reasonably low and stable then as well. However, I really encourage you to try and do cardio first thing in the morning. My A.M. cardio routine wakes me up and helps raise metabolism so that I stay in fat-burning mode for the rest of the day. I also credit it for helping me get over a plateau I reached when I was first trying to get in shape but couldn't drop that last bit of definition-obscuring fat. Once I added morning cardio to my routine, my abs stood out like never before.

There's a fat-burning bonus we all forget. I call it *hidden cardio*, and it's in plain sight if we just bother to look. Whenever possible, walk instead of ride, take the stairs even if the elevator is open and waiting for you, and pick the farthest parking spot at the grocery store. These little bonuses will show up in your exercise account. I think of it as "overweight protection," a little additional deposit that's there no matter what curves life throws at you. Even if it seems to be a small amount, it sure compounds fast. If you do just a little more than 100 calories a day worth of hidden cardio—without ruining it all at the snack bar—in a month you'll have vaporized a pound.

## STRENGTH TRAINING: LIFT WEIGHTS EVERY OTHER DAY

Lifting weights builds muscle, which not only makes you stronger but also helps make you lean. Remember, muscle is metabolically active and burns fat just to exist, even while we're sleeping. The more muscle we have, the more fat we burn, so by regularly working out with weights, we're priming our bodies to burn fat 24 hours a day, every day, 365 days a year. Muscles work miracles on our metabolism.

When it comes to weight training, the key words should be *short* and *intense*. The goal of lifting weights is to stimulate your muscles enough so that they'll regrow bigger and stronger but not to overstress them to the point of breakdown. The growth process occurs largely during rest periods.

When I first started working out, I listened to all that nonsense about how you had to work out every day to build muscle. Needless to say, I could have won the title of "Mr. Overtraining." I read the magazine profiles of various bodybuilders describing their grueling daily routines. Of course, what wasn't included in these write-ups was the fact that just about

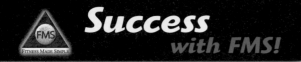
Dear FMS,

I'm 45 years old, and I have been battling weight problems since I graduated from high school in 1977. I had seen John's commercials several times prior to starting my program and they looked good to me, so I ordered two FMS videos to help me achieve my goals. I am 5'8½" tall, and when I started on the program, I weighed 225 pounds and had a 37-inch waist. My blood pressure was high (150/92) and so was my total cholesterol (220).

I started by watching and working out to John's videos until I had the workouts memorized. I used light weights at first and increased them over time. For cardio, I started walking two miles a day four days a week until I built up to my current three to four mile runs five to six days a week. I also started a low-carb, low-fat diet based on John's

every one of these guys was juiced up on chemical cocktails consisting of megadoses of anabolic steroids and other illegal, health-risking drugs. Since many of the muscle-building benefits of steroids are linked to their anticatabolic powers, they tend to lessen or prevent the muscle breakdown that occurs with overtraining. For the natural, health-conscious, and law-abiding weight trainer, following such a routine of overtraining will ultimately lead to substantial muscle mass *loss*.

That's why I want you to start by lifting weights every other day, about three or four days a week. I think it's best to focus on a different area of the body during each workout. In my plan you'll work your chest and back on one day, shoulders and arms on another, and legs on a third.

information and my own experiences over the years. Three months after I started the FMS program, my weight dropped to 180 pounds and my waist was down to 32 inches. Three months later I hit 165 pounds and my waist was 30 inches. My blood pressure was down to 118/70 and my total cholesterol was 188. At that time I started working out with more weight and have put on about eight pounds of muscle, bringing my weight to 172 pounds with my waist still at 30 inches.

My wife, family, and friends have been astonished by my results. Thanks again.

## AB TRAINING: FOUR OR FIVE TIMES PER WEEK

Just about everyone wants a defined midsection. Men usually desire the tight six-pack look of ripped abdominals. Women tend to look more for a toned, flat, cellulite-free stomach region. Whichever is your preference, both of these looks can be very difficult to achieve; that's why you don't see more amazing abs on the beach.

It's ironic to me that in this technological age where tons of ab videos and devices litter sporting goods stores and television screens, we don't see more chiseled midsections. I've tried various abdominal gadgets and gizmos in my own quest to see if I actually had abs, but for me, and apparently for many others, these pricey items just don't get the job done. Let me clarify that: they work fine to strengthen and develop the abs but don't necessarily produce the *definition* seen on the video cover models. That's because they only take into account one aspect of abdominal sculpting, and that's training.

Most people don't get the ripped results they want because they don't know that the secret to creating defined abdominals involves these two key points:

- **A smart nutrition program** that helps reduce naturally occurring fat deposits in our stomach areas so we can actually see the results of our exercise efforts. By following the FMS nutrition plan that I laid out in previous chapters, you'll go a long way toward making your abs show.
- **Variety in training routines** to stimulate ab muscle development. This can be done with or without expensive ab gizmos.

I'll go over the ab exercises I use to maximize muscle development in Chapter 9. I train my abs four or five days a week, and I rotate these exercises regularly. This variety keeps my muscles stimulated and growing by not allowing them to get used to just one routine. Each of these exercises can be done right at home, and the whole workout is only about 10 minutes long.

One other tip when it comes to building a six-pack: I suggest doing your ab work at night and putting your hand on your abs while you're training. This practice helps develop the mind-muscle connection, and knowing I don't want to end my day feeling a squishy layer of water and fat keeps me from overeating at the dinner table.

# CONSISTENCY: THE KEY TO SUCCESS

Here are two final things to keep in mind about exercise. First, make sure to get enough rest each night. It's one of the most overlooked factors in developing a successful fitness program. Muscles need rest to grow since we break down muscle fibers during exercise. Once fed proper nutrients, they rebuild bigger and stronger during rest periods. Not allowing yourself to rest leads to overtraining or, because you don't have enough energy, to no training at all. Being overtired or overtrained throws our bodies out of whack, depletes our energy, and robs us of control.

The second thing to remember is that fitness isn't stored—fat is stored. You have to keep it up, make the choice to put exercise in your life every day. Consistency is the key to getting results. Squeeze in 30 to 45 minutes of activity every day and you'll look and feel better than you ever thought possible.

## JOHN-ISM

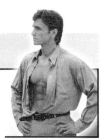

With fitness anything is possible. It creates a ripple effect and makes everything better—physically, mentally, and emotionally.

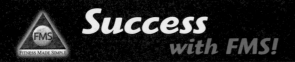
Dear John,

I just wanted to take the time to write and express my thanks for sharing your knowledge with us little people. Our results are based on our own discipline, but you have provided me an incredible foundation to work with.

I'm a 24-year-old Chinese male and, in my past, I've had difficulty understanding how to build up (especially my arms and chest) and trim down. It's difficult to afford a personal trainer, so I was at a loss for what to do. The fact of the matter is, if I had not learned from FMS, I might still be doing my exercises wrong and not understanding what is necessary to progress to the level I wanted. I read tips and other routines from magazines and websites, but alone they don't give you the details you really need.

FMS gave me great insight on the number of reps and variety of exercises to do. In fact, to my surprise, in my last workout I benched about 20 pounds more than my previous weight set. Results like that just keep the motivation going. Within the past month my shoulders have grown, my chest expanded, and my arms became rock hard with more mass. I must say it's been toughest for me to expand my arms . . . and now *finally!* My abs are more developed than I had really thought they could be. Honestly, I was extremely surprised the workouts from FMS did all this! I didn't use any of the machines I see people use so often, and

I literally just trained my abs 10 to 15 minutes a day every other day or so. Now, I can totally feel how rock hard they are.

Your insights on nutrition were also extremely helpful. I've gotten more in the habit of understanding what's in certain foods and watching what I eat. On the weekdays I stick to a pretty strict nutrition plan, but on the weekends I allow myself to indulge a little (lots of sushi, some pizza, etc.), kind of like a reward so I don't go crazy missing some of my favorite foods. Some of my friends think I'm nuts to be skipping out on certain foods on the weekdays, but I keep telling them that it's a plan for a goal. Doing this not only helps my devotion to bodybuilding but builds my commitment to other things. If I work hard to stick to these plans, I can apply the same concept to other variables in my life.

My friends have all complimented me and even my parents have been showing me off like, "Look at my son!" For my Chinese circle there are not many buff guys to go around. My gal friends are definitely impressed, and I've noticed stares in my direction from some workout situations. Even my martial arts buddy has complimented me on my arms now, and, coming from his standards, that actually means something. The best part was seeing one of my ex-girlfriends (still a friend) and she straight up said, "Geez, you look so good I almost regret letting you go!" That made my day!

I haven't reached my goal yet—which is to look like *you*! But someday! Nonetheless, it has been your workout ethic and insights that have helped me build a perfect foundation for myself. And with that I believe I can do more things I place my mind on!

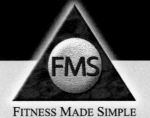

FITNESS MADE SIMPLE

# THE FMS WORKOUT PLAN

In this chapter I'll show you how to do all the exercises that will help you transform your body. I'll also give you a specific training plan you can follow. Remember, I believe failing to plan is planning to fail.

# JOHN-ISM

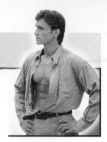

The first step to accomplishing
something is believing you can.

Here are some points to keep in mind:

- **Warm-ups.** It's important to warm up before you work out. I like to start
  with some yoga-based moves and stretches, which I'll show you in the
  following pages. The stretches feel great, get your blood flowing, and rev
  up your energy so you can have a great workout.

- **How much weight to use.** The amount will be different for every person. With each exercise you should use a weight you can lift anywhere
  from 8 to 12 times. I generally aim for 10 repetitions, but I make sure the
  10th one is a strain. You should almost need assistance on it. Once you
  can do the 10th rep easily, then you've got to challenge yourself again
  by increasing the weight next time.

- **Sets and reps.** For each exercise I recommend three sets of 8 to 12 reps.
  If you can't do this many at first, that's fine. Just try to do a little more
  each workout. Keep in mind that it doesn't matter where you start out.
  What counts is where you end up and that you enjoy the journey.

- **Rest periods.** The amount of time between sets depends on your goal. If
  your primary purpose is to lose fat, try to go from one set or exercise right
  to the next one. This practice will keep your heart rate up and help you stay
  in a fat-burning mode, but you may be able to handle only lighter weight
  for your 8 to 12 reps. If the goal is primarily to build muscle while using
  heavier weight, I like to rest about a minute between sets and exercises.

- **Form.** Avoid herky-jerky movements. Whatever the exercise is, use slow
  and controlled movements, concentrating on the concentric (contract-
  ing) motion as you're raising the weights and the eccentric motion as

you're lowering them back down. You should always be able to feel the stress on your muscles. If you keep the mind-muscle connection throughout your whole workout, you'll get the maximum results from your exercise time.

- **Variety.** Your body is an extremely complex, brilliant, adaptable mechanism. You can have the greatest workout plan in the world, but if you keep doing the same thing over and over again, your body will adapt to it and you'll start seeing diminishing returns on your exercise investment. That's why varying your routine is crucial. For each area of your body, I've included several exercises that you can pick and choose from during your workout. You can also add variety by changing your tempo. For instance, during one workout do a 3 count on the eccentric motion of the exercises and a 1 count on the concentric motion. During your next workout try a 1 or 2 count on each motion.
- **Home or gym.** The FMS plan includes home and gym versions of the strength workouts. They contain some different exercises, but either one will help you accomplish your goals of building muscle and losing fat. Choose whichever workout is more convenient for you.

## JOHN-ISM

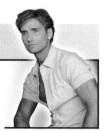

Fitness is not a game of how miserable you can make yourself. You have to make it part of your lifestyle—not something you tolerate but a part of it that you actually enjoy and look forward to.

You know what Fitness Made Simple has done for me. Your program is and has been my way of life. It's very inspirational to see all of your FMS commercials on television. You never stop motivating me to stay fit. The best part is that you keep things "real." You never try to sell a "quick fix" product that can be misleading to people. Being in the fitness industry myself for more than 10 years, I can say that FMS is the only legitimate program on the market as far as I'm concerned. FMS not only works but you make it so that it fits into people's lifestyles—no excuses.

As a personal trainer, nutrition consultant, and mother of two children, I completely support everything that you are promoting in your FMS program. My clients use Fitness Made Simple as their guide to happier and healthier lives. They have been attaining excellent results consistently now for years by following FMS. This is a win-win situation for us all, thanks to you.

Fitness Made Simple promotes wellness and lifestyle changes that will produce lifelong results. I believe any person at any level of fitness at any age, male or female, will succeed with this program. It's simple and it makes a lot of sense. Thank you for being my motivation!

FITNESS MADE SIMPLE

Note: you can see one of Maryann's clients, Rebecca, who follows the FMS principles, demonstrating some exercises with John in the following pages.

# WARM-UPS

Do five or six of the following stretches before your strength workout, focusing on:

- **Breathing.** Take deep cleansing breaths. Breathe in through the nose and out through the mouth or nose.
- **Slow movements.** Don't overdo it. Everything should be slow and controlled. Your body will slowly give in to the stretches and become more flexible.

## Neck Rolls

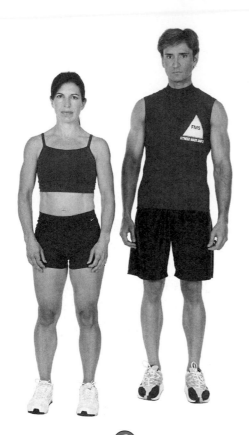

**1**

Stand with your feet shoulder-width apart and your hands at your sides.

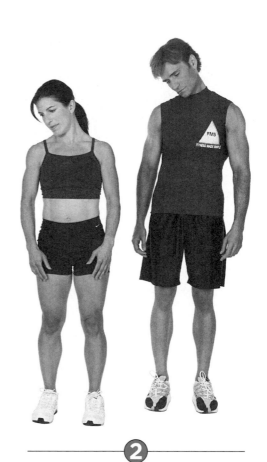

**2**

Drop your chin to your chest and then slowly rotate your head in a circular motion.

# Shoulder Rolls (Circles) Forward and Reverse

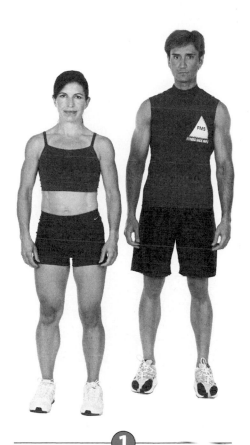

**1**

Stand with your feet shoulder-width apart and your hands at your sides.

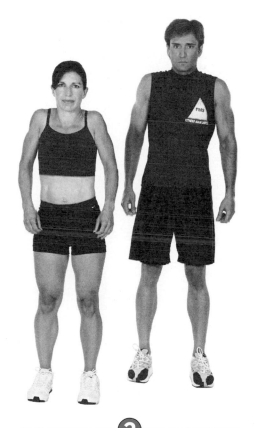

**2**

Keeping your arms straight, rotate your shoulders up and down in a circular motion.

## Shoulder Front and Back

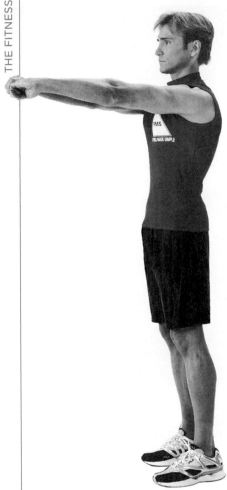
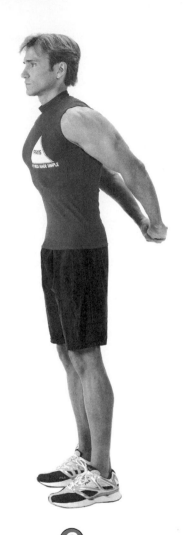

**①**

Stand with your feet shoulder-width apart. Hold your arms out in front of you at chest level and clasp your hands together. Pause, feeling the tension in your shoulders.

**②**

Now unclasp your hands, put your arms straight behind you, and clasp your hands behind your back, again feeling the tension in your shoulders. To add difficulty, bend forward at the waist. Repeat.

**126**

## Chest and Back Stretch

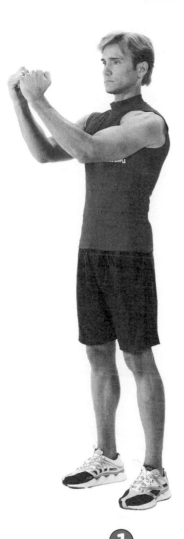

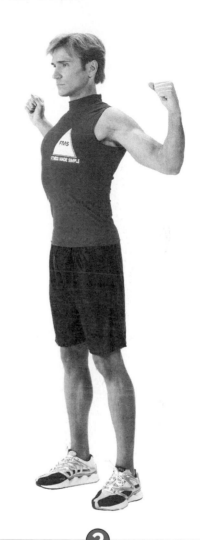

**1**

Stand with your feet shoulder-width apart. Bend your arms at the elbow and squeeze them together in front of you almost like you're hugging a barrel.

**2**

Keeping your arms bent, rotate them to each side. You should feel your back muscles contract almost like you're trying to hold a ball between your shoulder blades. Repeat.

## Around-the-World Chest Stretch

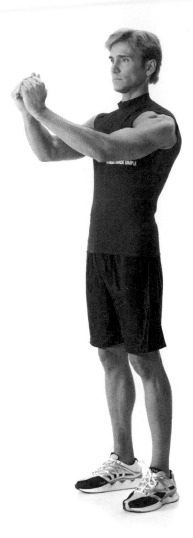

**1**

Stand with your feet shoulder-width apart. Bend your arms at the elbow and squeeze them together in front of you almost like you're hugging a barrel.

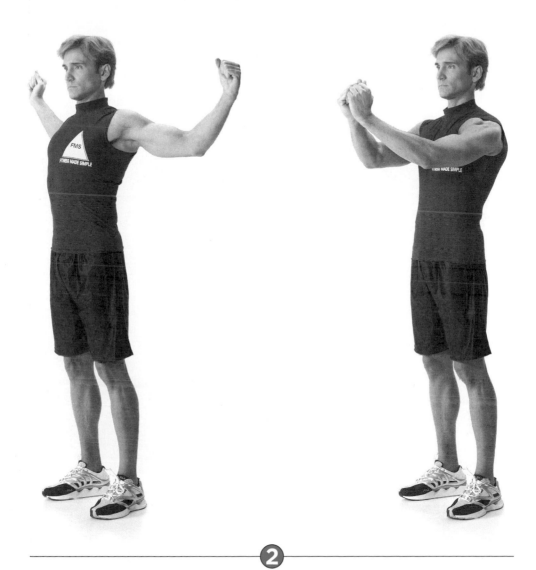

**2**

Bend your arms slightly and rotate them back in a wide motion.
You should feel your chest muscles opening up. Repeat.

## Reach for the Stars

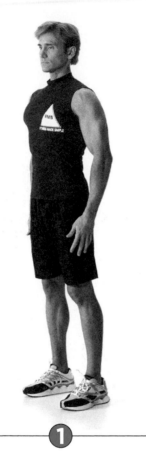

**①**

Stand with your feet shoulder-width apart.

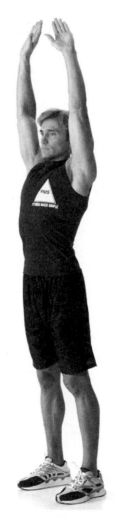

**②**

Raise your arms in the air and reach up as high as you can. Your feet are planted firmly on the ground as you reach to the sky. You're giving your body roots and wings.

## Crescent (Half-Moon) Stretch

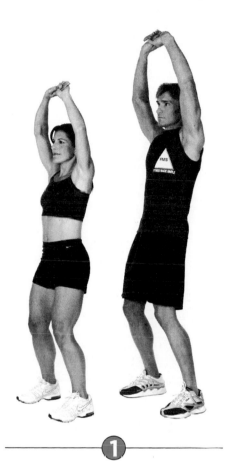

**1**

Stand with your feet shoulder-width apart. Clasp your hands together with your arms raised above your head.

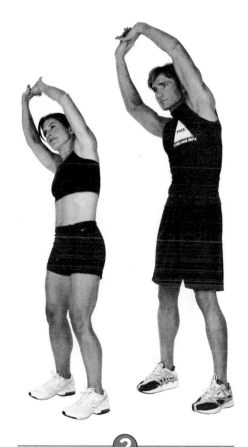

**2**

Bend your upper body in a crescent position to the right side. Feel the stretch throughout your entire upper body, particularly the lat muscles in your back. Repeat on the left side.

## Swan Dive to Waterfall/Lower Back Stretch

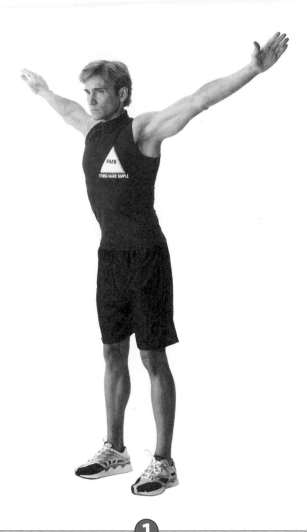

①

**Swan Dive:** Spread your arms like wings and descend by bending at the waist.

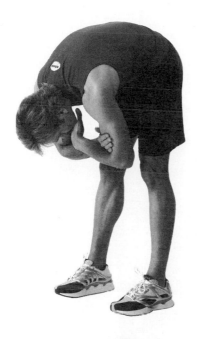

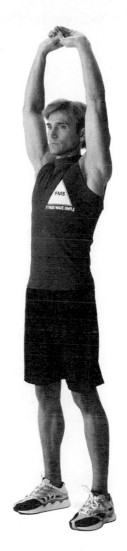

**②**

**Waterfall/Lower Back Stretch:**
To stretch your lower back a little, wrap your arms together and just hang a bit (about 8 to 10 seconds) while feeling your back muscles stretching. Let the muscles relax. Surrender to the stretch. You can also grasp the back of your calves or ankles and hold to further stretch the back.

**③**

Put your hands on your knees and roll your back up slowly as if you're arching it like a cat. Reach for the stars and arch back. Go back down to waterfall and repeat.

THE FITNESS TRIANGLE

## Triangle Pose and Side/Waist Stretch

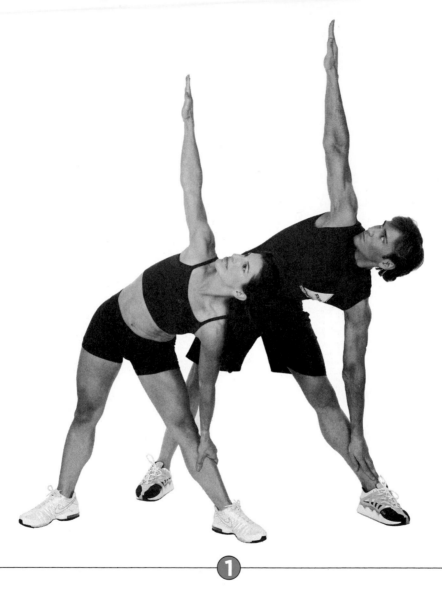

**1**

Put your left hand on your left shin and reach up with your right hand. This is called Triangle Pose. Reach to the sky, keeping your eyes on your thumb.

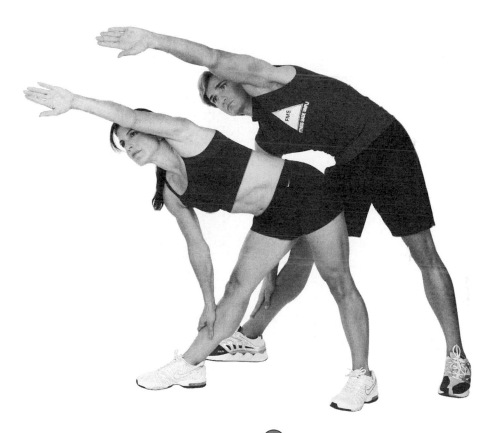

**2**

Reach over with your left arm to really stretch your lat muscles.
Repeat on the other side. As you get more flexible, you can reach
farther down your leg or even touch the floor. It increases the
difficulty and maximizes the stretch.

## Wide Leg Squats

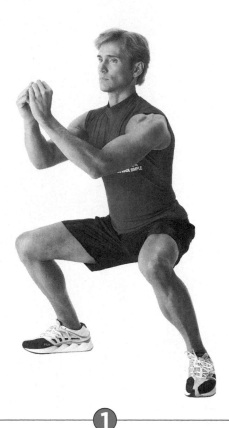

**1**

Stand with your feet a little farther than shoulder-width apart and your toes pointing out.

**2**

Keeping your back straight, bend your knees and lower your butt as close to the floor as you can.

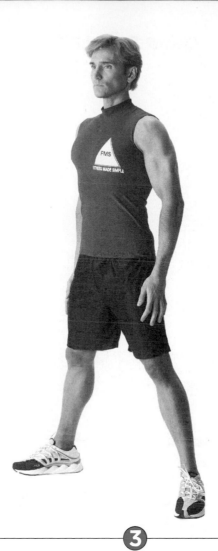

**3**

Squeezing with your glutes and thighs, return to the standing position.

## Quad Stretch

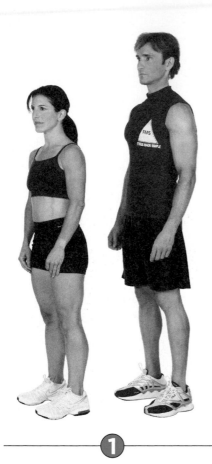

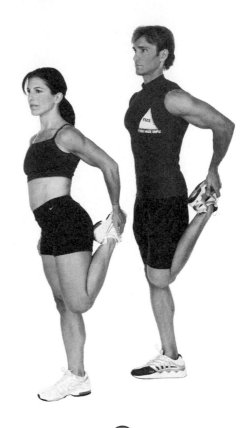

**1**

Stand with your feet shoulder-width apart.

**2**

Bend your left leg behind you and grasp it with your left hand. If necessary, hold on to the top of a chair or the wall for support. Pause, feeling the stretch in your thigh. When you get used to balancing on one leg, you can increase the difficulty by putting your right arm forward or up. This helps you feel the stretch even more. Repeat with your right leg.

## Hamstring Stretch

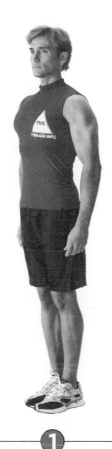

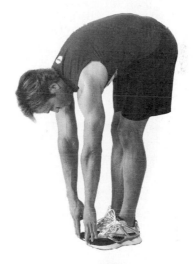

**1**

Stand with your feet together.

**2**

Reach down to touch your toes, holding that position for 3 counts. Then come up and go back down. Try to keep your legs straight and feel the stretch right down the entire back of your thighs. If you can't keep your legs perfectly straight, bend them slightly and then try to straighten them as much as you can as you go along. Don't bounce.

139

## Inner Thigh Stretch, Runner's Stretch, and Warrior/Exalted Warrior

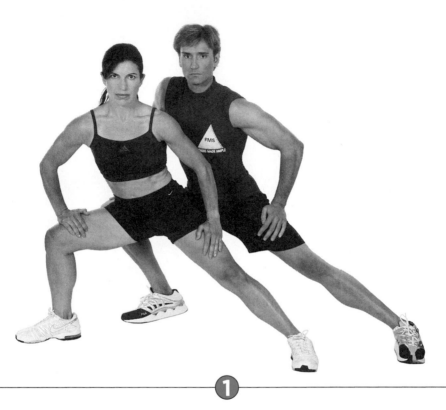

**1**

**Inner Thigh Stretch:** Turn your right leg outward a little and stretch your inner thigh, keeping your right knee over your ankle. Feel the stretch throughout the inner part of your left leg.

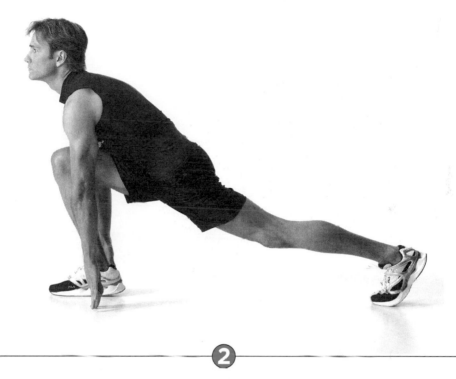

**2**

**Runner's Stretch:** Now turn to the right and bring your hands to the floor to stretch out the backs of your legs. Repeat on the left side.

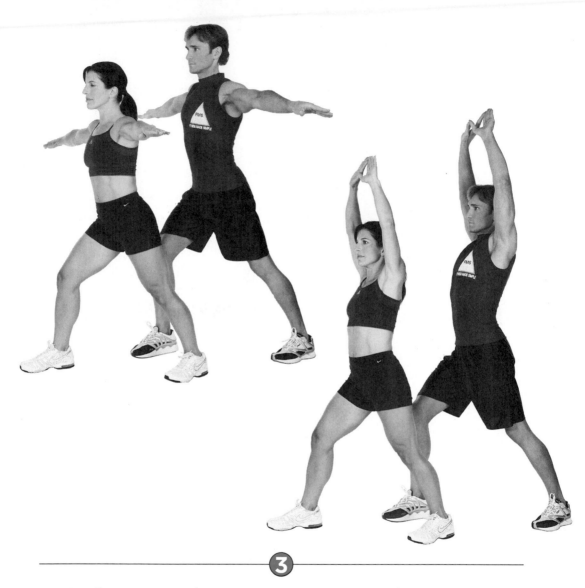

**3**

**Warrior/Exalted Warrior:** For variety, and to add a little more "power yoga" into the mix, go up to the Warrior Pose with arms parallel to the floor and then to the Exalted Warrior Pose with arms above head.

# THE WORKOUTS

## The FMS Seven-Day Exercise Planner

Here's a breakdown of how the FMS Workout Plan looks over the course of a week. Remember, since your goal is to do a weight workout every other day, you'll do three weight workouts the first week and four the following week.

Don't worry if you can't do all of the exercises I recommend at first. Your goal is progress, not perfection. Just do what you can today and strive for a little more tomorrow.

| | DAY 1 | DAY 2 | DAY 3 | DAY 4 | DAY 5 | DAY 6 | DAY 7 |
|---|---|---|---|---|---|---|---|
| **A.M.** | Cardio | Cardio | Cardio (optional) | | Cardio | | Cardio |
| **Any time** | | Chest/ Back | | Shoulders/ Arms | | Legs | |
| **P.M.** | Abs | | Abs | | Abs | | Abs |

# DAY 1

**A.M.** Cardio

As discussed in previous chapters, first thing in the morning before you have breakfast is the best time to perform your cardio workout. Any low-impact exercise is fine—elliptical trainer, stationary bike, treadmill, walking, or even running around the block a few times. Work your way up to 40 to 50 minutes per session. Aim for an intensity that lets you carry on a conversation without losing your breath.

**P.M.** Abs Workout

In the evening do five abdominal Power Minutes in succession: during each Power Minute you perform a single abdominal exercise until a minute has elapsed. Try to mix upper/mid abdominal exercises, lower ab exercises, and oblique exercises in each workout.

## Standard Crunch

*(targets upper/mid abdominals)*

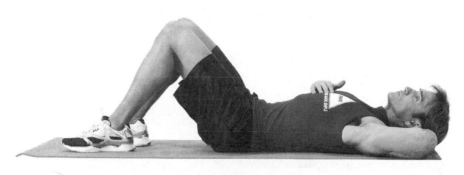

**①**

Lie on your back with your knees bent, feet resting either on the floor or on a bench, and either one or both hands behind your head. I put one hand on my abs to feel the contraction and keep the mind-muscle connection.

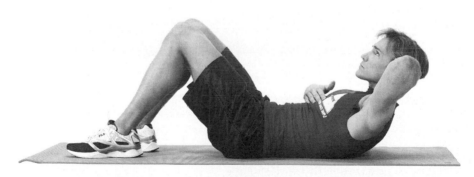

**②**

Crunch up, bringing your shoulder blades off the ground. Pretend there's a string attached to your upper torso, pulling it up while your lower back is stuck to the ground.

## Oblique Crunch

*(targets obliques)*

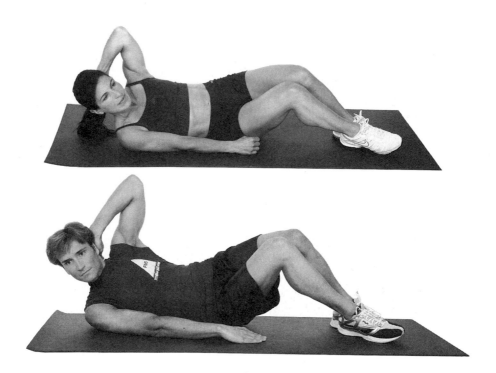

**1**

Lie on your right side with your legs on top of each other and your knees bent. Place your left hand on the side of your head, covering your left ear.

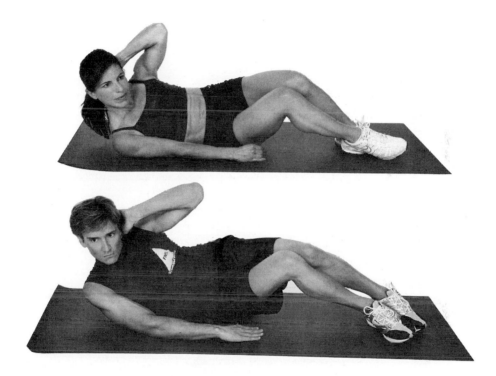

**2**

Crunch your side as high as you can, focusing the movement to work the obliques as much as possible. Pause. Then return to the starting position. Perform for 30 seconds on the left side, then repeat for 30 seconds on the right side.

## Ab Scissors

*(targets upper/mid and lower abdominals)*

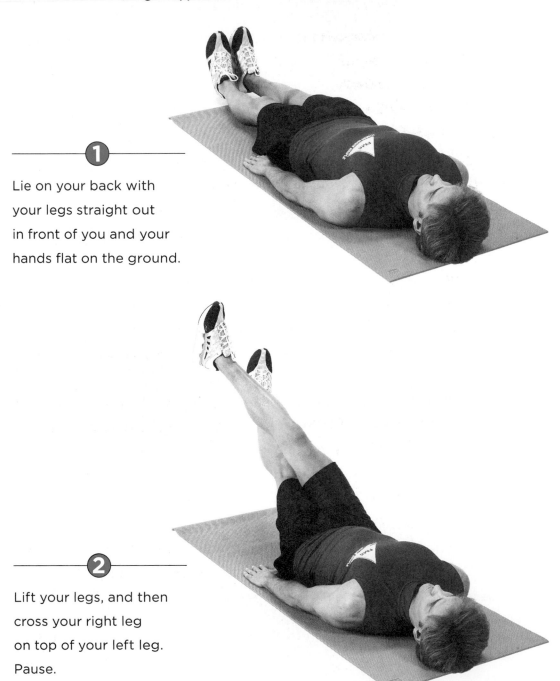

**1**

Lie on your back with
your legs straight out
in front of you and your
hands flat on the ground.

**2**

Lift your legs, and then
cross your right leg
on top of your left leg.
Pause.

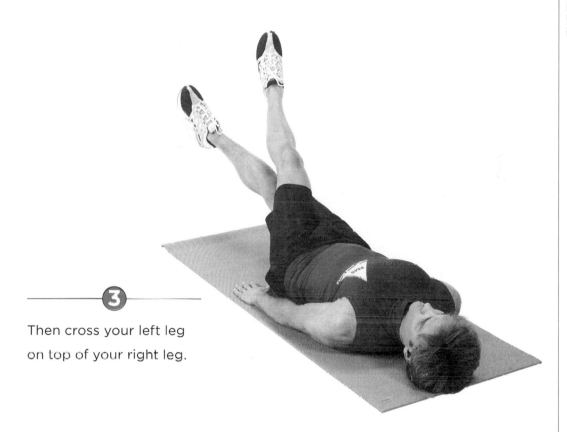

**3**

Then cross your left leg
on top of your right leg.

## Lower Ab Rockers

*(targets lower abdominals)*

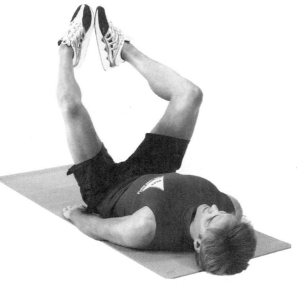

**1**

Lie on your back with your
head slightly off the ground,
your feet lifted, and your arms
at your sides on the mat.
Touch your toes together
and stick your knees out,
forming a diamond shape.

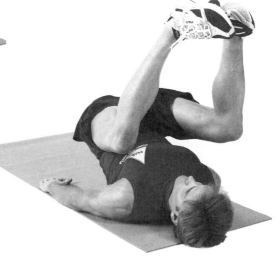

**2**

Rock forward, lifting your butt
off the ground while feeling
the squeeze in your lower ab
region. Pause. Then return to
the starting position.

## Alternate Bicycle

*(targets upper/mid abdominals and obliques)*

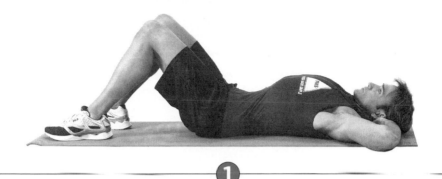

①

Lie on your back with your knees bent 90 degrees and your hands behind your ears.

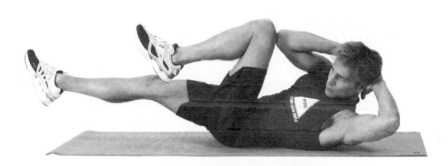

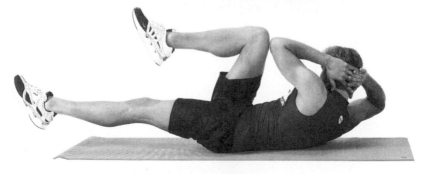

②

Pump your legs back and forth, bicycle style, as you rotate your torso from side to side by moving your elbow toward the opposite knee.

# DAY 2

**A.M.** | **Cardio**

Aim for 40 to 50 minutes of your favorite cardio exercise.

## Chest Workout (Home Version)

Do three exercises each workout, rotating your choice of exercises for variety.

## Flat Bench Press

*(three sets of 10–12 reps)*

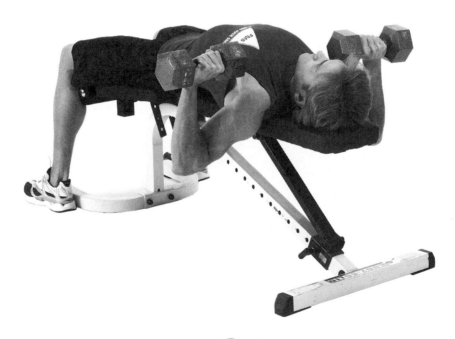

**1**

Lie on a flat bench holding a pair of dumbbells just above and outside your chest. Your feet should be flat on the floor for stability, your back and head firm against the bench.

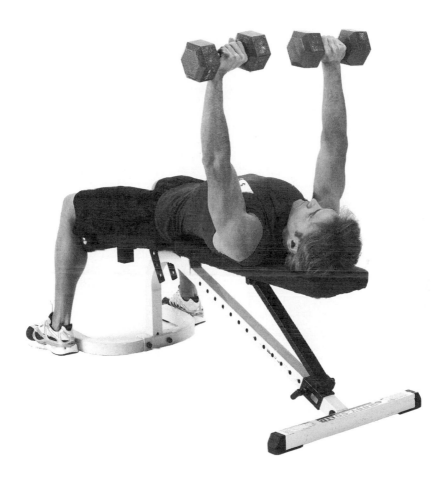

**2**

Push the weights up in a slanting motion so they almost meet when your arms are extended. Pause. Slowly lower them back to the starting position.

# Incline Press

*(three sets of 10–12 reps)*

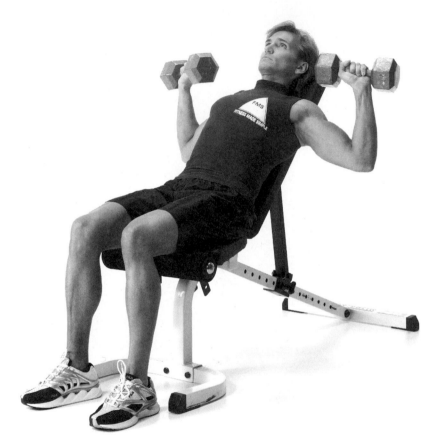

**①**

Lie on an incline bench (I prefer a 45-degree angle) holding a pair of dumbbells just above and outside your chest. Your feet should be flat on the floor for stability, your back and head firm against the bench.

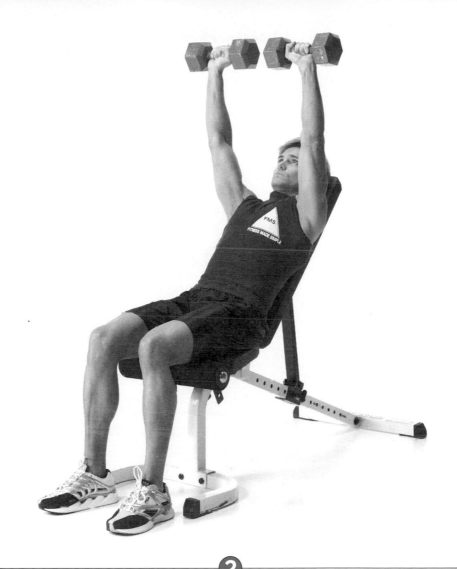

②

Push the weights up in a slanting motion so they almost meet when your arms are extended. Pause. Slowly lower them back to the starting position.

# Incline Fly

*(three sets of 10–12 reps)*

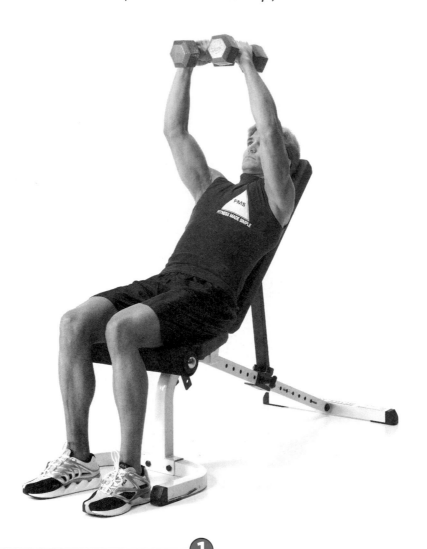

①

Lie on an incline bench with your feet planted firmly on the floor. Hold the dumbbells over your chest with your palms facing each other, arms extended, and elbows slightly bent.

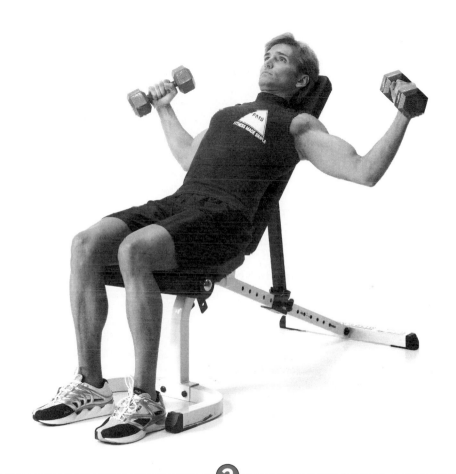

**2**

Slowly lower the dumbbells in an arc motion until your upper arms are parallel to the floor and your palms face the ceiling. Pause. Then lift the dumbbells along the same arcs to the starting position. Imagine that you're hugging a barrel.

## Push-Ups
*(three sets of 10–12 reps)*

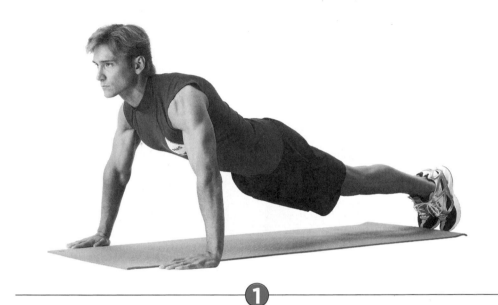

**1**

Get in push-up position with your hands shoulder-width apart.

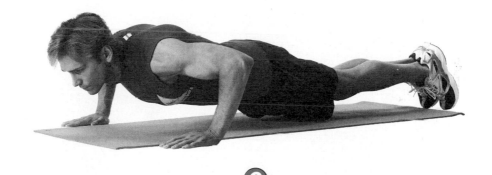

Bend at the elbows while keeping your back straight until your chin almost touches the floor.

## VARIATIONS

Do a different variation each workout. Push-ups work the chest and back along with the arms. Beginners can do what's called knee push-ups, with their knees on the ground, or standing push-ups against a wall. I do additional reps of push-ups if I'm not doing any other weighted exercises that day.

*Diamond-grip:* Put your hands together, forming a diamond with your thumb and fingers.

*Wide-stance:* Put your hands wider than shoulder-width apart.

*Close-grip:* Put your hands parallel to each other with your thumbs touching.

## Back Workout (Home Version)

Do both exercises each workout.

# Bent-Over Row
*(three sets of 10–12 reps)*

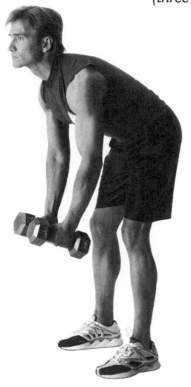

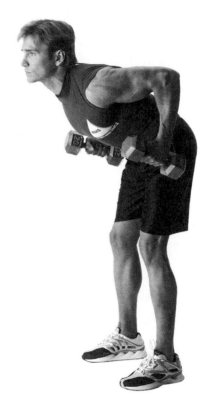

**1**

Stand with your knees slightly bent and legs shoulder-width apart. Bend forward so that your back is almost parallel to the floor. Holding a dumbbell in each hand, let your arms hang toward the floor.

**2**

With your palms facing in, pull the dumbbells toward you until they touch the outside of the chest. Pause. Then return to the starting position.

# Single Arm Rows

*(three sets of 10–12 reps)*

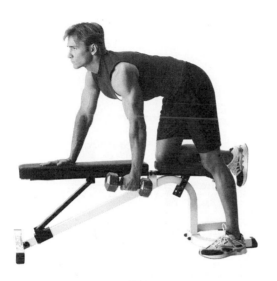

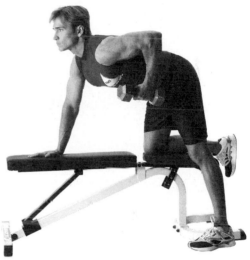

**①**

Hold a dumbbell in one hand as you place your opposite hand and knee on a weight bench. Your back should be flat and parallel to the bench. Let your arm hang straight down from your shoulder as you grip the dumbbell with your palm facing in.

**②**

Pull the weight straight up toward the side of your abdomen, finishing with your elbow pointing toward the ceiling. Pause. Then slowly lower the weight back to the starting position. When you finish all your reps with one arm, do the same number of reps with the other arm.

## Chest Workout (Gym Version)

Do these three exercises each workout.

# Flat Bench Press with Barbell

*(for variety use dumbbells as shown in the home version)*

*(three sets of 10–12 reps)*

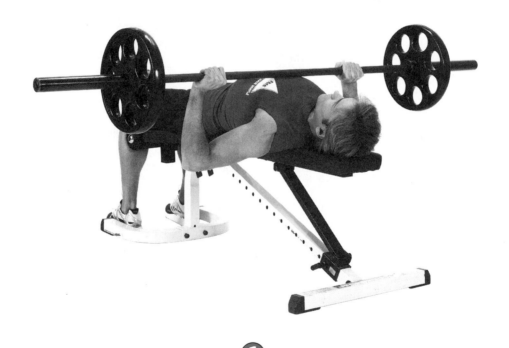

**1**

Lie on your back on a flat bench with your feet on the floor. Grasp the barbell with an overhand grip, placing your hands just beyond shoulder-width apart.

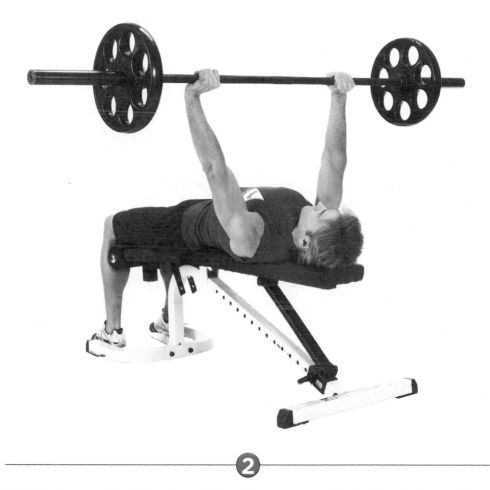

2

Lift the bar and hold it at arm's length over your chest. Slowly lower the bar to your chest. Pause. Then push the bar back to the starting position.

## Incline Press with Barbell

*(for variety use dumbbells as shown in the home version)*

*(three sets of 10–12 reps)*

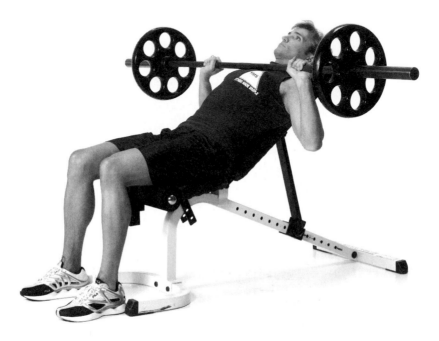

**1**

Lie on your back on a incline bench (I prefer a 45-degree angle) with your feet on the floor. Grasp the barbell with an overhand grip, placing your hands just beyond shoulder-width apart.

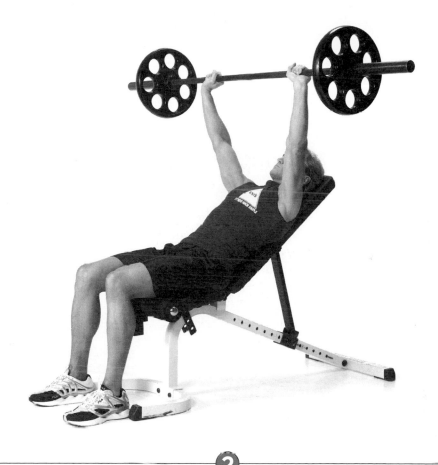

② 

Lift the bar and hold it at arm's length over your chest. Slowly lower the bar to your chest. Pause. Then push the bar back to the starting position.

## Cable Crossover

*(three sets of 10–12 reps)*

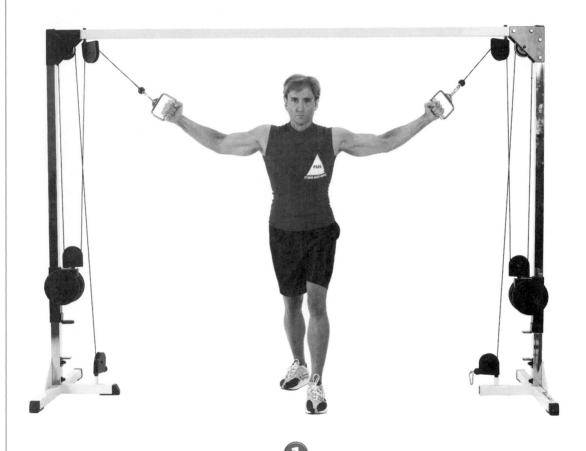

**1**

Stand inside a cable crossover with the stirrup handles attached to the high pulleys.

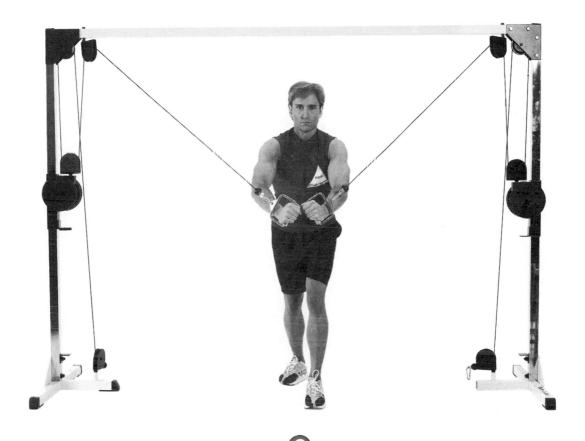

②

Slightly bend your knees and use your chest to bring your arms down until they meet in front of your body. Pause. Then return the weights to the starting position.

## Back Workout (Gym Version)

Do three exercises each workout, rotating your choice of exercises for variety.

# Bent–Over Barbell Row

*(three sets of 10–12 reps)*

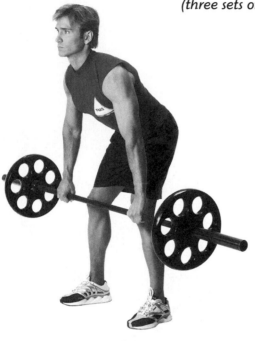

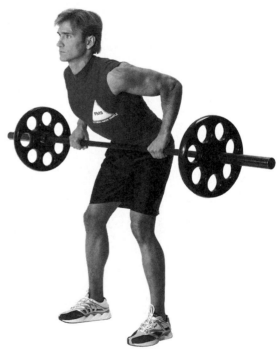

**1**

Grasp a barbell with an overhand grip that's just beyond shoulder-width and hold it at arm's length. Stand with your feet shoulder-width apart and knees slightly bent. Bend at the hips until your torso is at a 45-degree angle and let the bar hang straight down from your shoulders.

**2**

Pull the bar up to your torso. Pause. Then slowly lower it.

## Lat Pull-Down

*(three sets of 10–12 reps)*

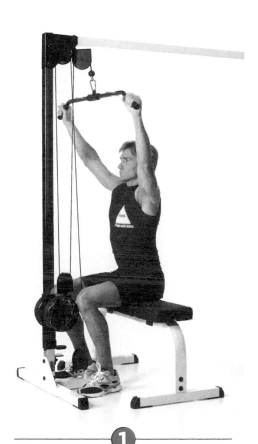

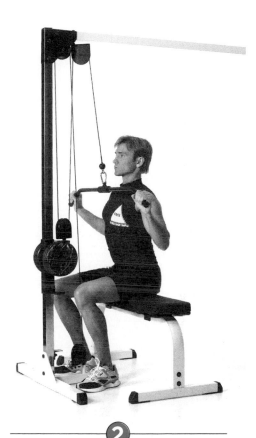

**①**

Stand facing a lat pull-down machine. Reach up and grasp the bar with an overhand grip that's slightly wider than your shoulders. Sit on the seat, letting the resistance of the bar extend your arms above your head.

**②**

Pull the bar down until it touches your upper chest. Pause. Then return to the starting position.

# Lat Pull-Up

*(three sets of 10–12 reps)*

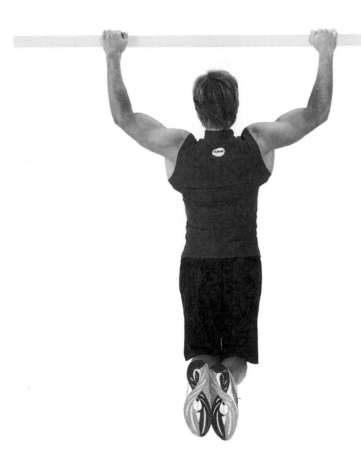

**1**

Grasp a chin-up bar or lat pull-up bar with an overhand grip and your hands more than shoulder-width apart. Hang from the bar with your arms completely extended, your knees bent, and your feet behind you.

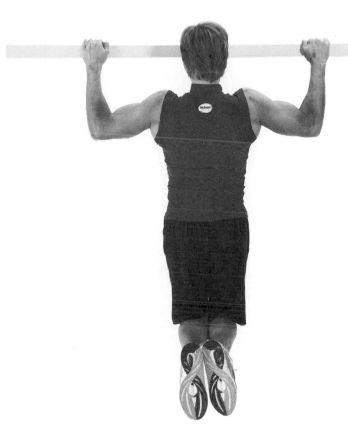

**2**

Pull yourself up until your chin rises above the bar. Pause. Then return to the starting position.

## Cable Row

*(three sets of 10–12 reps)*

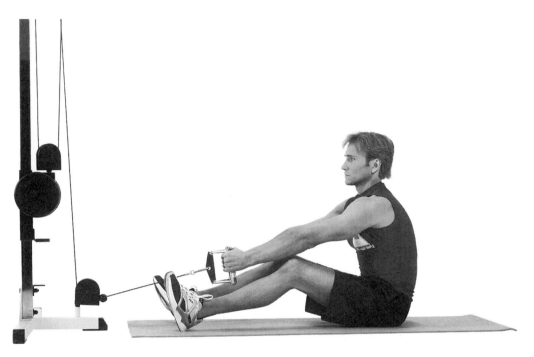

1

Attach a stirrup handle (or straight bar) to the low cable. Sit and grab the handle. Your torso should be upright, your shoulders should be back, and your arms should be almost straight in front of you.

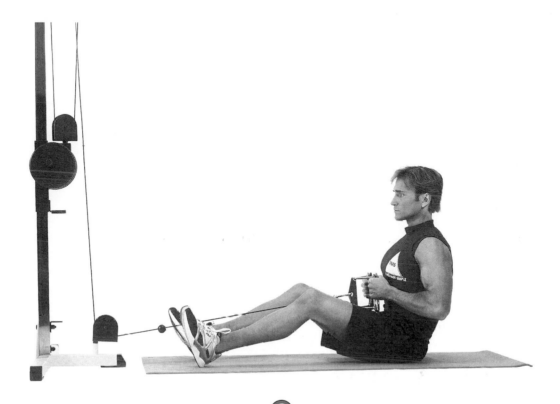

**2**

Pull the handle to your midsection. Pause. Then slowly return to the starting position.

# DAY 3

### A.M. Cardio (optional)

The cardio workout is optional. Particularly if you're just starting to exercise, you may want to use today as a rest day and allow your body to recover.

### P.M. Abs Workout

In the evening do five abdominal Power Minutes in succession: a single abdominal exercise until a minute has elapsed.

## Standard Crunch

*(targets upper/mid abdominals)*

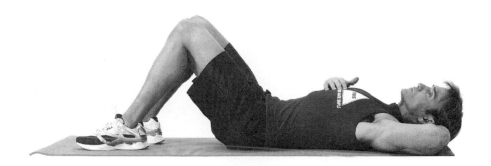

**①**

Lie on your back with your knees bent, feet resting either on the floor or on a bench, and either one or both hands behind your head. I put one hand on my abs to feel the contraction and keep the mind-muscle connection.

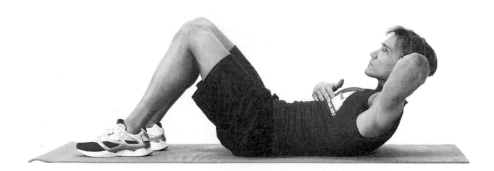

**②**

Crunch up, bringing your shoulder blades off the ground. Pretend there's a string attached to your upper torso, pulling it up while your lower back is stuck to the ground.

## Trunk Twist

*(targets lower obliques)*

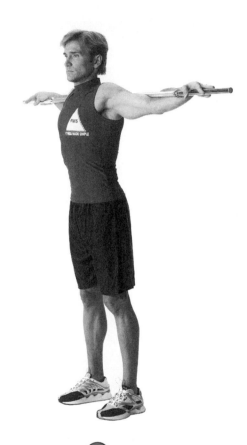

**1**

Grasp a bar or stick and place it behind your neck. Stand with your knees bent and feet shoulder-width apart.

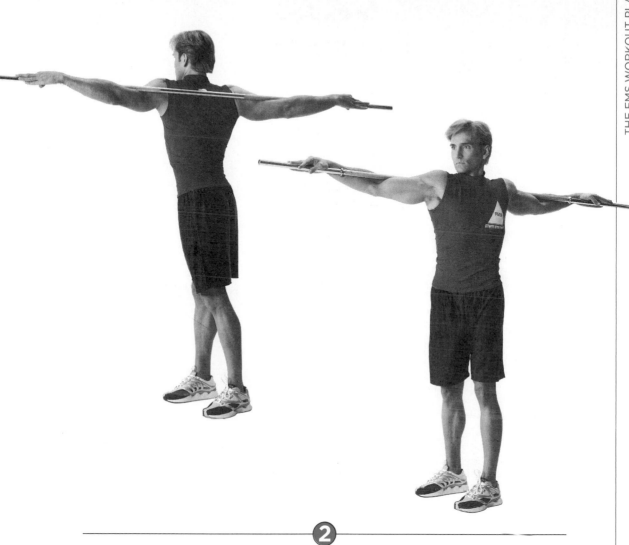

**2**

Keeping your hips stationary, twist to the right as far as you can in a slow, controlled motion and then twist back to your left as far as you can, feeling the twist in your oblique muscles. Continue the exercise for one minute.

# V Crunch

*(targets lower abdominals)*

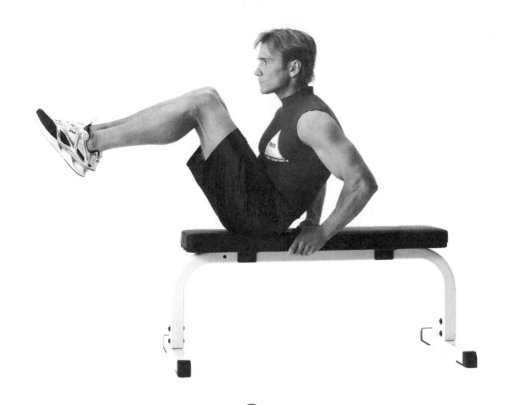

**①**

Sit on the edge of a bench with your knees folded into your chest.
Hold on to the sides of the bench to support yourself.

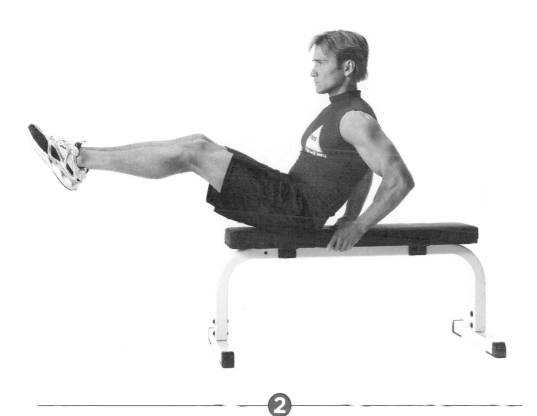

**2**

Extend your legs straight out in front of you. Pause. Then return to the starting position.

## Superman Stretch

*(targets upper/mid and lower abdominals)*

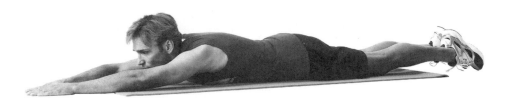

**①**

Lie down on your abdomen and extend your arms out in front of you.

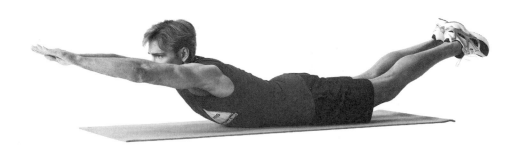

**②**

Raise your arms and legs slightly off the floor while feeling the squeeze in your lower back region. You should now be in a Superman flying position. Hold this stretch for 10 to 20 seconds at a time. Pause. Repeat.

## Lying Leg Raises

*(targets upper/mid and lower abdominals)*

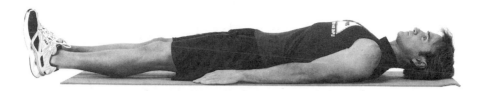

**1**

Lie on your back with legs straight.

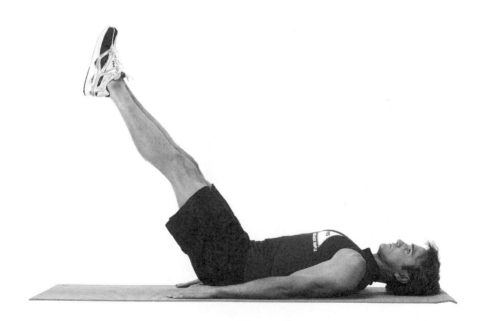

**2**

Keeping your lower back pressed against the floor, raise your legs to a 45-degree angle. Pause. Then slowly lower them.

# DAY 4

## Shoulders Workout (Home Version)

Do three exercises each workout, rotating your choices for variety.

## Military Press
### (three sets of 10–12 reps)

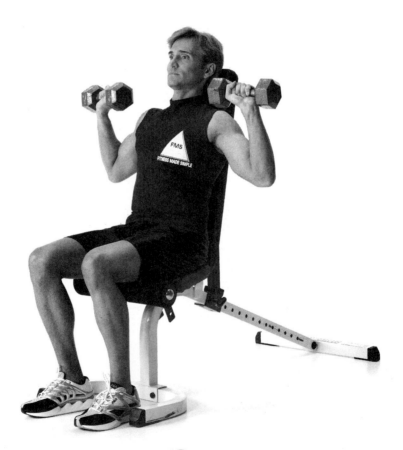

**1**

Sit on a bench or chair, holding one dumbbell in each hand, about level with your ears.

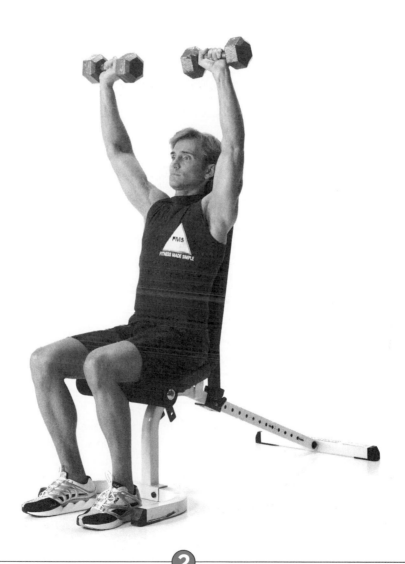

②

Push the dumbbells straight overhead so that your arms are almost fully extended. Pause. Then return to the starting position.

## Frontal/"Zombie" Raises

*(three sets of 10–12 reps per arm)*

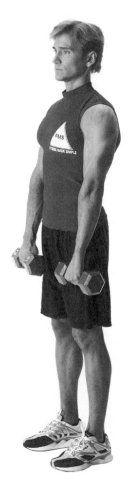

Grab a pair of dumbbells and stand with your feet shoulder-width apart. Hold the dumbbells down at arm's length in front of your legs, with your palms turned toward your thighs. Bend your elbows slightly.

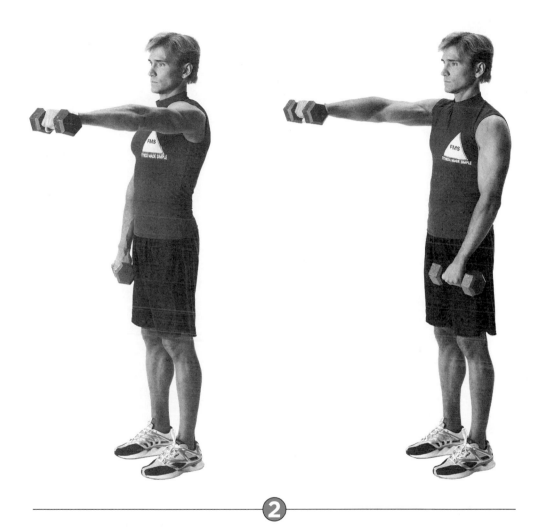

**2**

Lift the dumbbells, alternating arms one at a time, straight up in front of you to about shoulder level. Pause. Then slowly lower them to the starting position.

# Lat Raises

*(three sets of 10–12 reps)*

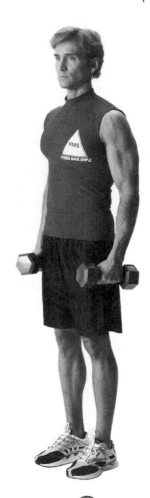

### ①

Stand and hold a pair of dumbbells down at arm's length with your palms facing your sides.

### ②

Keeping a slight bend in your elbows, raise the weights out to your sides until your upper arms are parallel to the floor. Pause. Then slowly return to the starting position.

# Bent-Over Rear Deltoid Raises

*(three sets of 10–12 reps)*

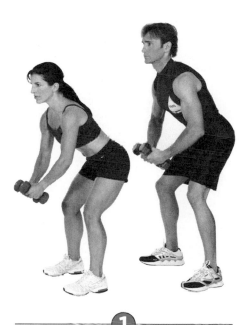

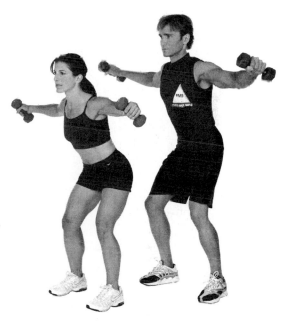

**①**

Grab two dumbbells and stand with your feet slightly more than shoulder-width apart and your knees slightly bent. Bend over at the hips, holding the dumbbells in front of you with your arms hanging straight down, palms facing each other, and elbows slightly bent. The dumbbells should be an inch or two apart.

**②**

Raise the dumbbells up and out to your sides until your upper arms are parallel to the floor. Pause. Then lower the dumbbells slowly to the starting position.

## Biceps Workout (Home Version)

Do two exercises each workout, rotating your choices for variety.

## Standing Dumbbell Curls

*(three sets of 10–12 reps per arm)*

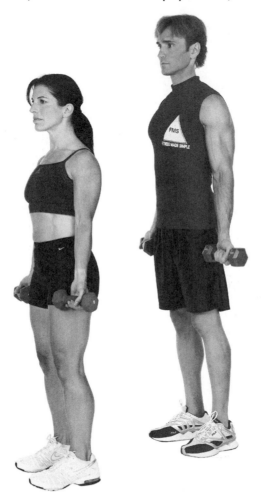

①

Grab a pair of dumbbells and stand with your feet shoulder-width apart. Hold the dumbbells down at arm's length in front of your legs with your palms facing away from you.

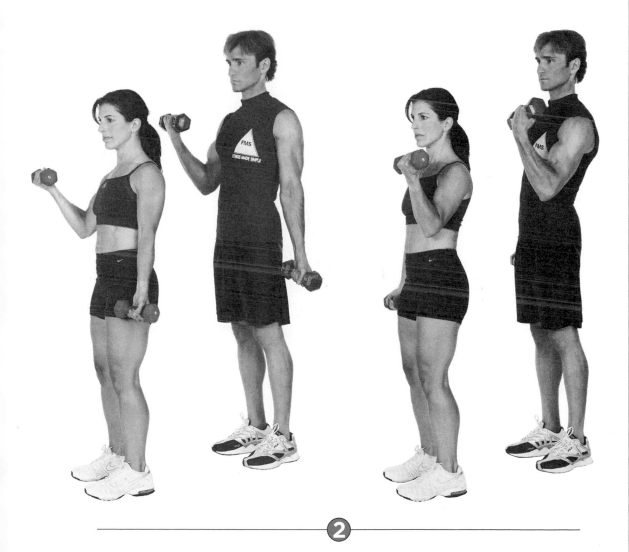

**2**

Curl the weights toward your shoulders, alternating arms one at a time, hold for a second, and then return to the starting position.

## Hammer Curls

*(three sets of 10–12 reps per arm)*

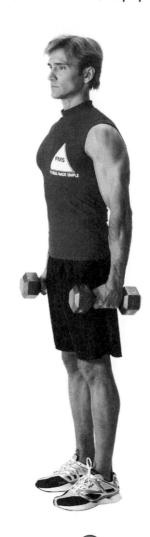

①

Grab a pair of dumbbells and stand with your feet shoulder-width apart.
Grasp the dumbbells with palms facing each other as if you
were holding a hammer in each hand. You can also do hammer curls
while seated.

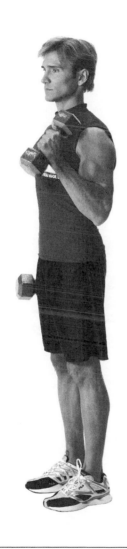
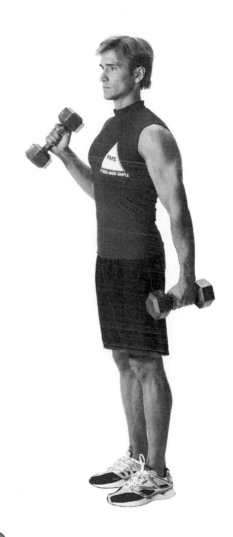

**2**

Curl the weights toward your shoulders, alternating arms one at a time, hold for a second, and then return to the starting position.

## Seated Alternate Dumbbell Curls

*(three sets of 10–12 reps per arm)*

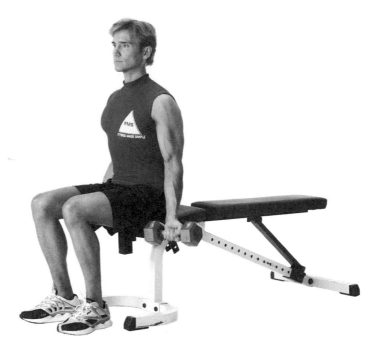

①

Sit on the end of a bench, holding a pair of dumbbells at arm's length with your palms facing out.

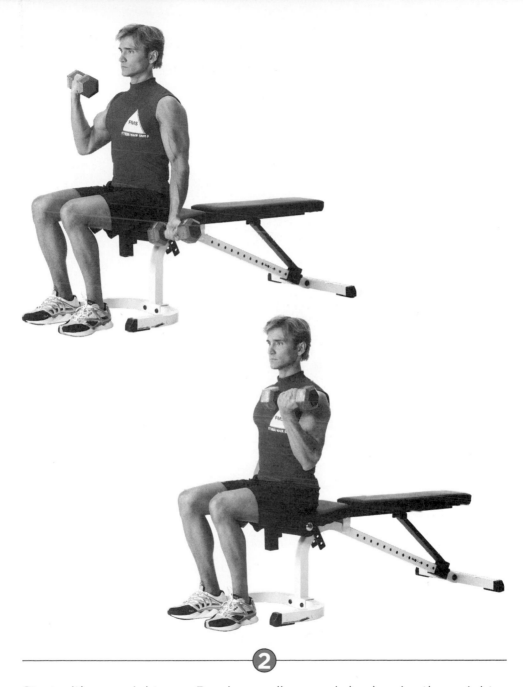

②

Start with your right arm. Bend your elbow and slowly raise the weight as high as you can without allowing your elbow to move forward. Pause. Then slowly return to the starting position. Alternate arms.

## Concentration Curls

*(three sets of 10–12 reps per arm)*

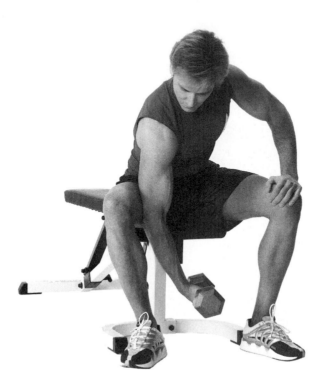

**1**

Sit at the end of a bench holding a dumbbell at arm's length between your thighs. With the back of your working arm resting against your inner thigh on that same side, lean forward at the waist and brace yourself with your nonworking arm on your opposite thigh.

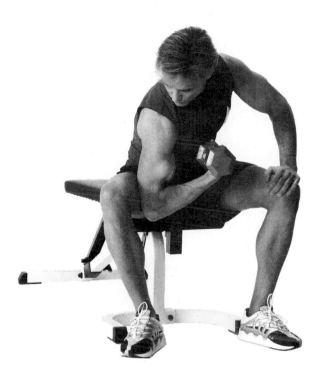

**2**

Hold this position as you curl the weight up as high as you can toward your chest. Pause. Then lower and repeat. Alternate arms.

Do two exercises each workout, rotating your choices for variety.

# Chair Dips
*(three sets of 10–12 reps)*

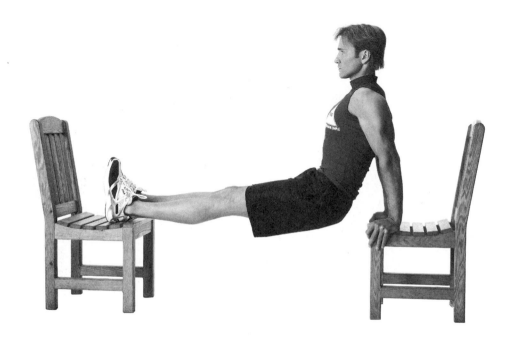

**1**

Place two chairs facing each other. Sit on one chair with your hands palm down and gripping the edge of the chair. Place your heels on the edge of the other chair and hold yourself up using your triceps.

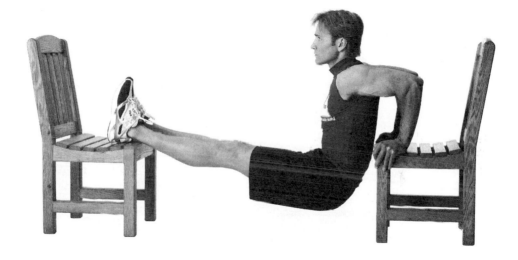

2

Dip down just far enough so that your behind clears the edge of the chair and lower yourself so your elbows are at 90 degrees. Push back up to starting position.

## Single Arm Triceps Extension

*(three sets of 10–12 reps per arm)*

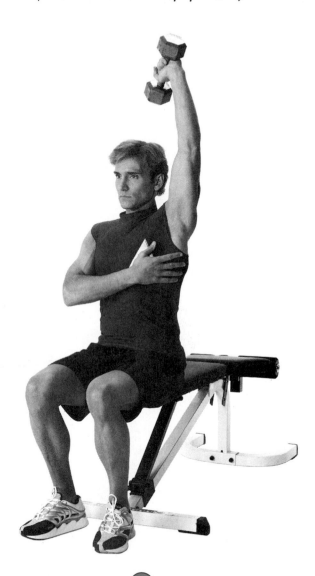

**1**

Sit on a bench holding a dumbbell over your head, supporting your working arm with your free arm.

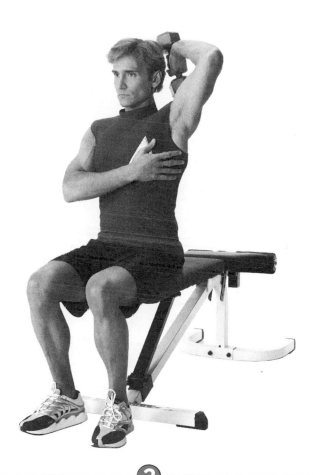

**2**

Lower the dumbbell until it's just above the base of your neck. Pause. Then press the weight back up to the starting position. Repeat with the other arm.

## Triceps Kickback

*(three sets of 10–12 reps per arm)*

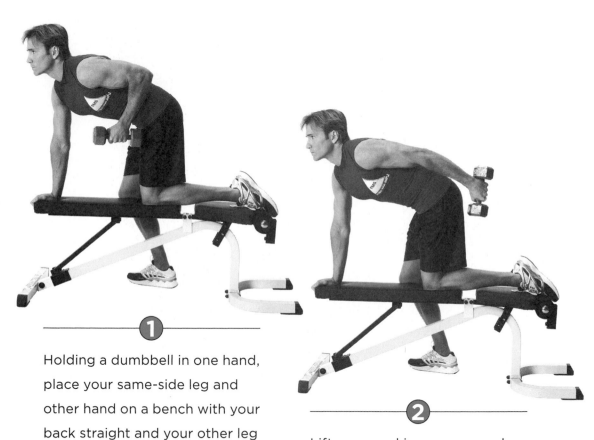

**1**

Holding a dumbbell in one hand, place your same-side leg and other hand on a bench with your back straight and your other leg on the floor.

**2**

Lift your working arm up and tuck to your side as you extend the dumbbell back until your arm is straight and parallel to the floor. Pause. Then lower and repeat. Keep the motion slow and controlled.

## French Press

*(three sets of 10–12 reps)*

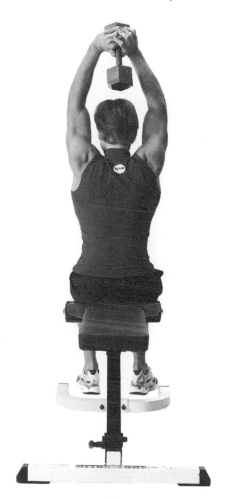

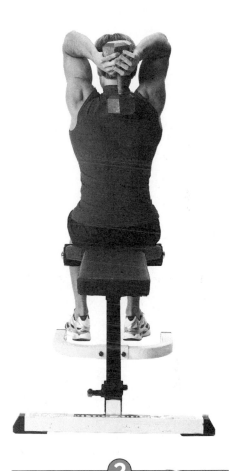

**1**

Grab a dumbbell and sit on a bench. Raise the dumbbell straight overhead so your palms face each other.

**2**

Without moving your upper arms, bend your elbows to slowly lower the weight behind your head. Pause. Then raise back to the starting position. Keep your elbows in close to your head to really target the triceps.

## Shoulders Workout (Gym Version)

In addition to the following exercises, the free-weight exercises shown in the home version can also be used in the gym. Do three exercises each workout. Rotate your choices for variety.

## Seated Military Press
*(three sets of 10–12 reps)*

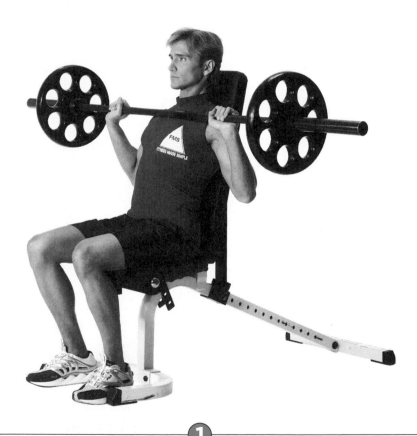

① 

Grab a barbell with an overhand grip, keeping your hands shoulder-width apart. While seated hold the barbell at shoulder level in front of you with your feet shoulder-width apart and knees bent.

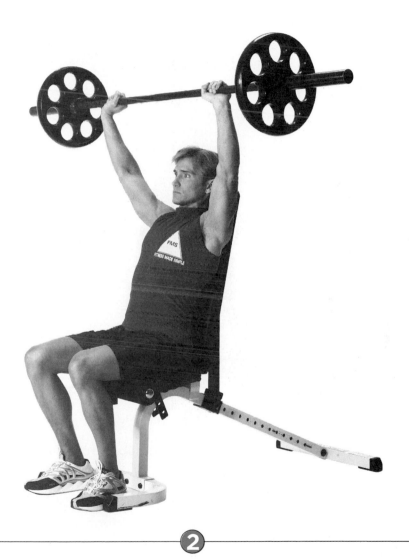

**2**

Push the weight straight overhead, leaning your head back slightly but keeping your torso upright. Pause. Then slowly lower the bar back to the starting position.

## Lat Raises (Machine)

*(three sets of 10–12 reps)*

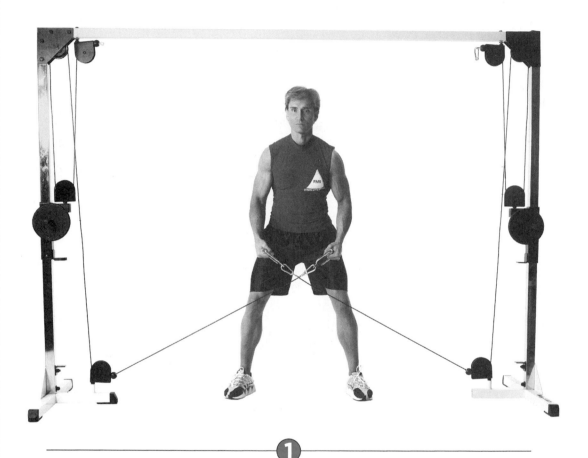

**1**

Stand slightly bent over in the center of the cable crossover apparatus so that your shoulders are lined up with the two sides of the machine. Grasp the right handle in your left hand and the left handle in your right hand. The wires attached to the handles should form an X.

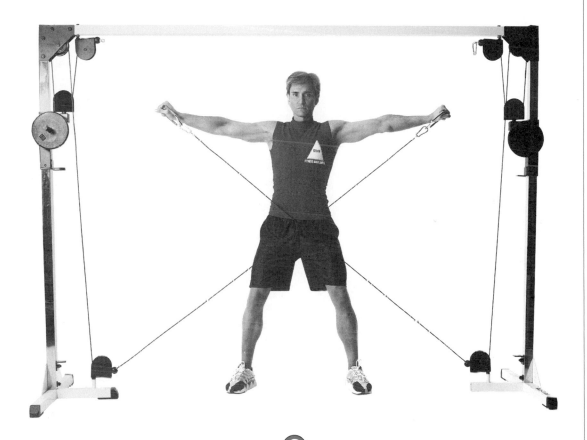

**2**

Extend your arms, pulling the weights up until your arms are parallel to the floor. Concentrate on feeling the contraction in the lateral, or side, muscles of your shoulders.

# Upright Rows
*(three sets of 10–12 reps)*

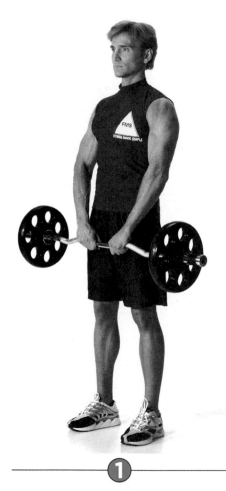

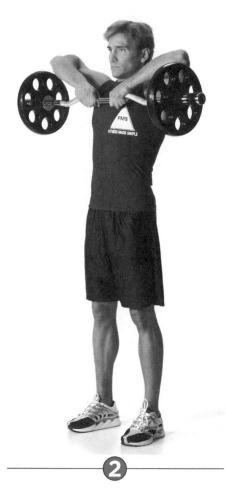

**①**

Stand upright with your knees slightly bent. Hold a barbell at arm's length against the front of your thighs with an overhand grip, keeping hands shoulder-width apart.

**②**

Pull the bar up to your chest until your upper arms are parallel to the floor. Pause. Then return to the starting position.

## Biceps Workout (Gym Version)

Do two exercises each workout, rotating your choices for variety.

# Standing Barbell Curls

*(three sets of 10–12 reps)*

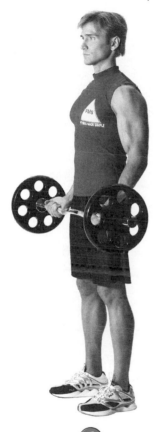

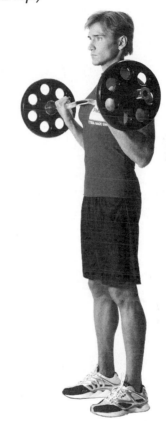

**①**

Grab a barbell with an underhand grip, keeping your hands just beyond shoulder-width apart. Stand upright with your knees slightly bent and hold the bar down at arm's length in front of your thighs.

**②**

Pull the bar to your chest by bending your elbows. Raise the weight as high as you can without allowing your elbows to move forward. Lower the bar to the starting position.

## Seated Alternate Dumbbell Curls

*(three sets of 10–12 reps per arm)*

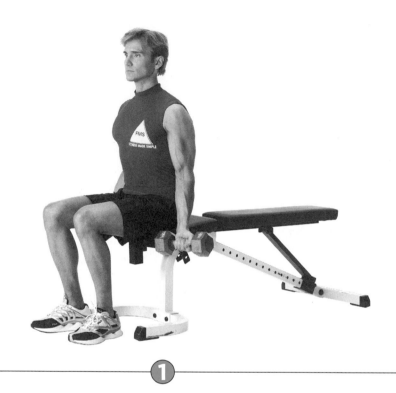

①

Sit on the end of a bench, holding a pair of dumbbells at arm's length with your palms facing out.

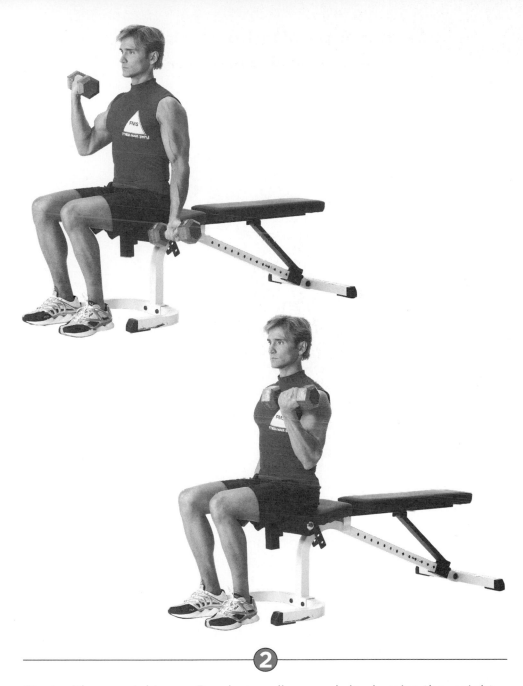

②

Start with your right arm. Bend your elbow and slowly raise the weight as high as you can without allowing your elbow to move forward. Pause. Then slowly return to the starting position. Alternate arms.

## Concentration Curls

*(three sets of 10–12 reps per arm)*

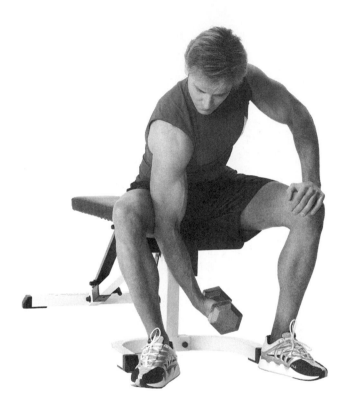

**①**

Sit at the end of a bench holding a dumbbell at arm's length between your thighs. With the back of your working arm resting against your inner thigh on that same side, lean forward at the waist and brace yourself with your nonworking arm on your opposite thigh.

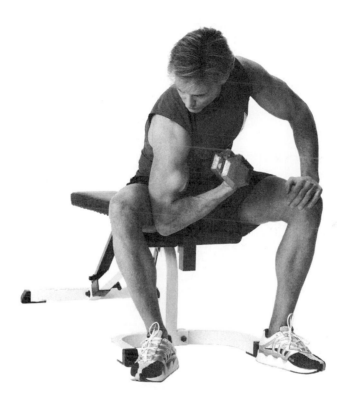

**2**

Hold this position as you curl the weight up as high as you can toward your chest. Pause. Then lower and repeat. Alternate arms.

## Triceps Workout (Gym Version)

Do two exercises each workout, rotating your choices for variety.

## Triceps Pushdown
*(three sets of 10–12 reps)*

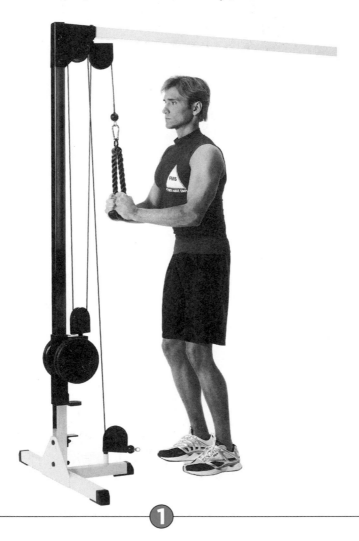

**1**

Stand in front of a cable station with a bar or rope handles attached to a high pulley. Grasp the bar or rope with both hands. Keep your knees bent, your back straight, and your upper arms close to your torso.

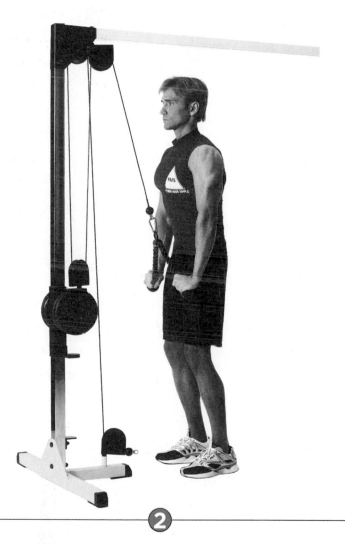

**2**

Extend your arms down from your chest toward the floor until they're straight. Pause. Then return to the starting position.

# Lying Triceps Extension

*(three sets of 10–12 reps)*

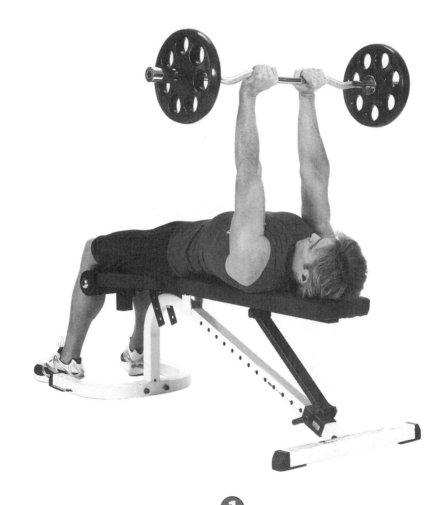

①

Grab an EZ-curl bar and lie back on a bench, holding the bar straight up over your chest.

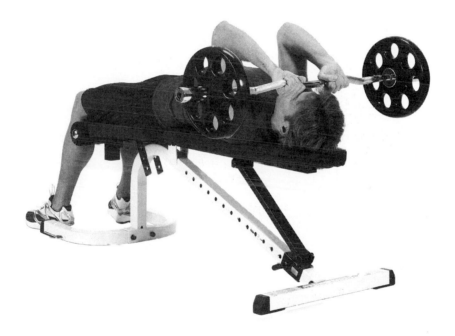

**2**

Slowly lower the bar to your forehead or just behind it. Pause. Then push back to the starting position. Keep your elbows in to really target the triceps.

## French Press

*(three sets of 10–12 reps)*

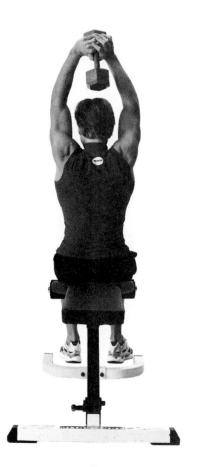

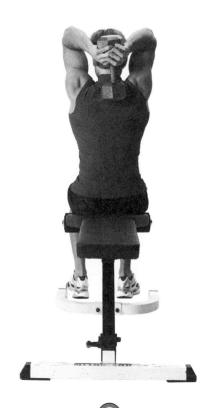

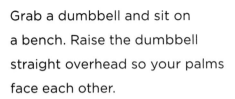

**①**

Grab a dumbbell and sit on a bench. Raise the dumbbell straight overhead so your palms face each other.

**②**

Without moving your upper arms, bend your elbows to slowly lower the weight behind your head. Pause. Then raise back to the starting position. Keep your elbows in close to your head to really target the triceps.

# DAY 5

**A.M.** Cardio

Aim for 40 to 50 minutes of your favorite cardio exercise.

**P.M.** Abs Workout

Repeat the abs routine from day 1.

# DAY 6

## Legs Workout (Home Version)

Do all four exercises each workout.

## Dumbbell Squats
### *(three sets of 10–12 reps)*

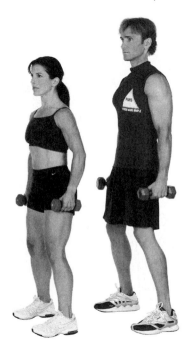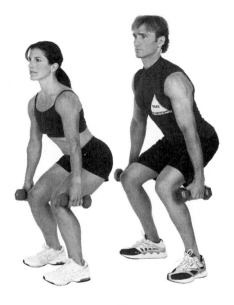

Grab a pair of dumbbells and hold them down at arm's length at your sides. Set your feet shoulder-width apart, with your knees slightly bent, back straight, and eyes focused straight ahead.

Slowly lower your body as if you were sitting into a chair, keeping your back in its natural alignment and lower legs nearly perpendicular to the floor. When your upper thighs are parallel to the floor, pause, and then return to the starting position. This exercise really hits the thighs and glutes.

## Stiff-Legged Dead Lift

*(three sets of 10–12 reps)*

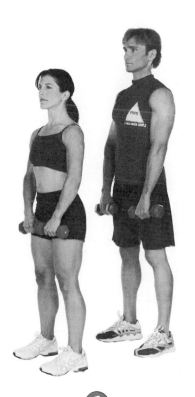

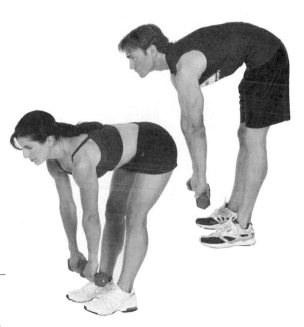

**①**

Stand holding a pair of dumbbells, palms facing toward you, with your arms hanging down in front of you.

**②**

Keeping your back straight, slowly bend at the hips as you lower the dumbbells close to the floor. Squeeze your glutes and hamstrings and return to the starting position.

## Dumbbell Lunges

*(three sets of 10–12 reps per leg)*

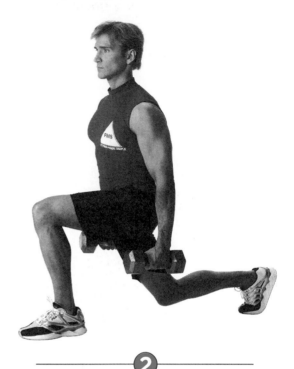

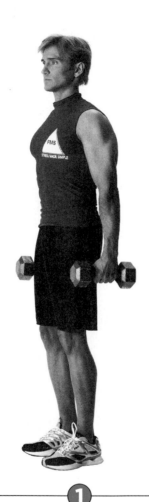

**1**

Grab a pair of dumbbells and hold them down at your sides. Stand with your feet hip-width apart.

**2**

Step forward with your nondominant leg (e.g., your left leg if you're right-handed) and lower your body until your front knee is bent 90 degrees and your rear knee nearly touches the floor. Your front lower leg should be perpendicular to the floor and your torso should remain upright. Push yourself back up to the starting position as quickly as you can and repeat with your dominant leg.

## Standing Calf Raises

*(three sets of 20–30 reps; I find calves are particularly hard to build and require more stimulation to develop)*

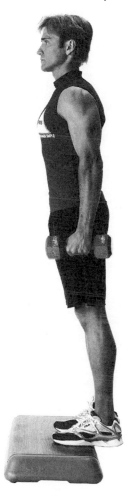 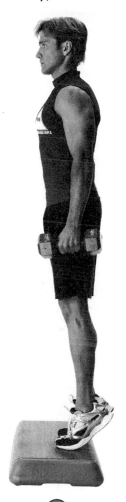

**1**

Stand on the balls of your feet on a step or block while holding a dumbbell in each hand at your sides.

**2**

Lower your heels as far as you can, and then rise up on your toes as high as you can. Pause. Feel the squeeze in your calf muscles. Then repeat the full range of motion.

221

## Legs Workout (Gym Version)

Do four exercises each workout, rotating your choices for variety.

## Leg Extensions
*(three sets of 10–12 reps)*

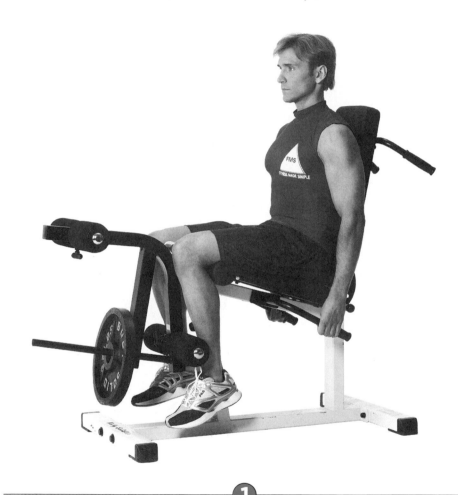

**①**

Sit in a leg extension machine with the leg pad just above your ankles.

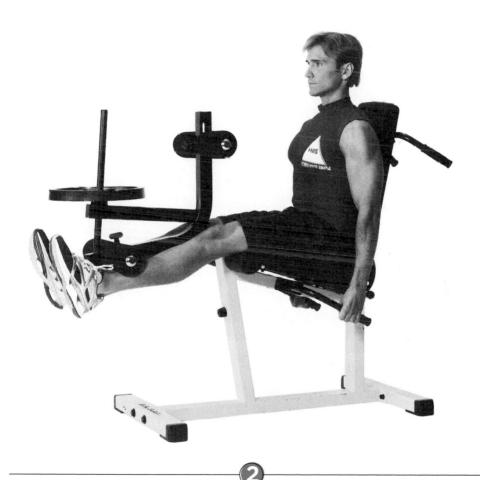

Extend your legs up until they're parallel to the floor. Pause. Then return to the starting position.

## Squats (Free Standing or Smith Machine)

*(three sets of 10–12 reps)*

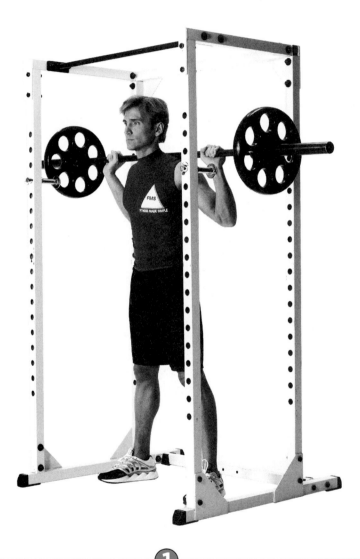

①

Place a barbell across your shoulders and step back from the squat rack. Set your feet shoulder-width apart and place your hands on the bar just beyond shoulder-width apart.

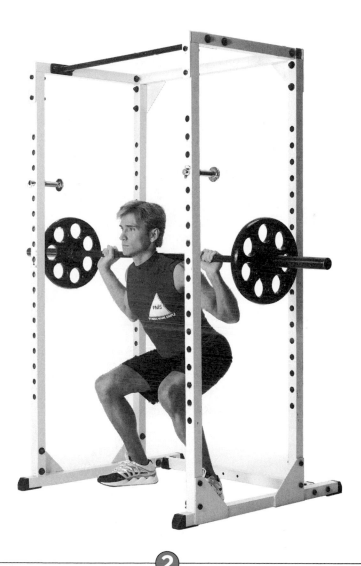

2

Bend at the knees and hips as if you were sitting in a chair and lower your body until your thighs are parallel to the floor. Pause. Then return to the starting position.

## Leg Press

*(three sets of 10–12 reps)*

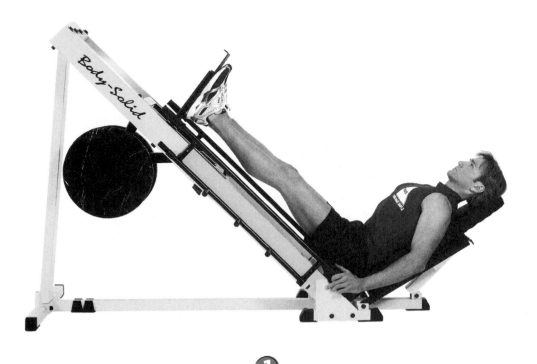

**1**

Sit in the leg press machine with your back against the pad and your feet on the force plate.

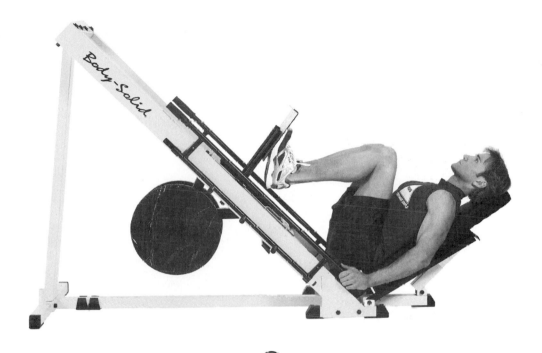

Release the safety lever and lower the weight slowly until your lower legs are parallel to the ground. Pause. Then push the weight up and return to the starting position.

## Calf Extensions

*(three sets of 20–30 reps; I find calves are particularly hard to build and require more stimulation to develop)*

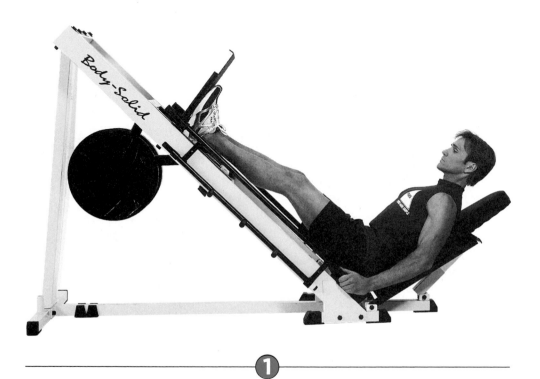

**1**

Sit in the leg press machine with your back against the pad and your feet on the force plate.

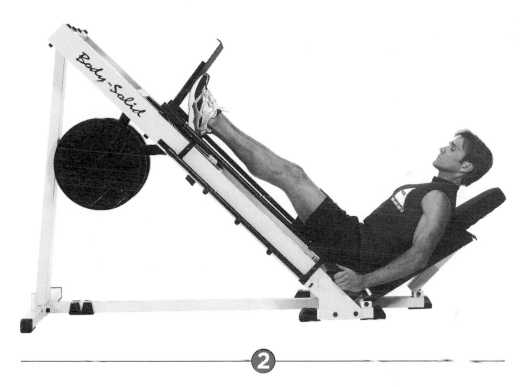

②

Without releasing the safety lever, push the force plate up with the balls of your feet, feeling the contraction in your calf muscles. Once your feet are fully extended, pause and then return to starting position.

# Leg Curls

*(three sets of 10–12 reps)*

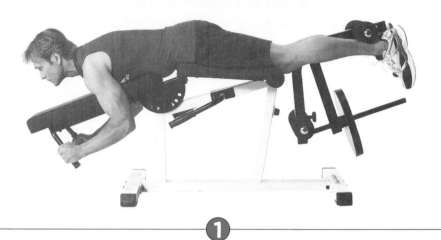

**①**

Lie on your stomach on the hamstring curl machine with the leg pad hitting you just above the Achilles tendons.

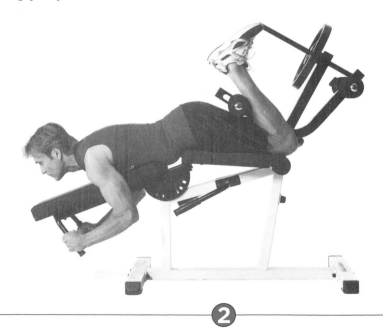

**②**

Curl the weights up until your feet get slightly behind your knees, almost touching your behind. Pause. Then return to the starting position.

# DAY 7

**A.M.** Cardio

Aim for 40 to 50 minutes of your favorite cardio exercise.

**P.M.** Abs Workout

Repeat the abs routine from day 3.

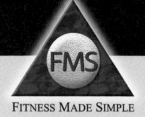

FITNESS MADE SIMPLE

# SUPPLEMENTS
## MADE SIMPLE

The third and final leg of the fitness triangle is supplementation. As I said earlier, however, it's not an equal of the other two. Remember my construction analogy from Chapter 2? Building your body is like building a house. The workout and nutrition sides of the fitness triangle are your foundation and walls. The supplement side is your furniture, paintings, and accessories. You can't hang a painting before you first erect a wall.

That's why I don't really recommend jumping on the heavily advertised supplement bandwagon until you already have the basic building blocks of an effective workout and meal plan in place. Too many people think supplements are the key to everything. They use them as a crutch—*pop a pill and you're on your way to a better body.* This type of thinking is just plain stupid. Some, and I emphasize *some*, supplements can help to enhance results or increase the effectiveness of your fitness program but, as the word implies, they're only *supplements* and not *substitutes* for proper nutrition and short, intense workouts.

When those other two sides of the triangle are in place, however, the addition of an effective fat-burning or muscle-building supplement can help speed and maximize the results of your gym and kitchen efforts. They're also great for renewing your enthusiasm and overcoming plateaus in a fitness routine.

I've tried practically every pill and potion out there, and I want to share with you some of the supplements that have helped me most over the years. Before we get to that, though, let me offer some more cautionary words about supplements in general.

## THE TRUTH ABOUT THE SUPPLEMENT INDUSTRY

As anyone who's picked up a bodybuilding or exercise magazine knows, the pages of these publications are littered with slick ads pushing everything from simple protein bars to high-tech-sounding insulin mimickers. They all promise to be the answers to our muscle-building and fat-burning dreams. These same products line the shelves of health food and vitamin stores in such variety that choosing one can be confusing, to say the least. Unfortunately, as I've found out through numerous, costly personal experiences, the majority of these pills and potions do more to lighten our wallets than to decrease our waistlines.

One reason is that the supplement industry is weakly regulated. Let me assure you, what's on the labels of these products is *not* always what's in the bottles. Many companies can get away with packaging impure or inferior products that go unchecked until someone does a laboratory analysis. For instance, a manufacturer can write that a protein powder contains 20 grams of high-quality whey protein per serving when its product may have only 10 grams of low-grade protein. The only way we as consumers would find out about this misrepresentation is if a detailed lab analysis was done. For me, choosing supplements is a trust game. That's why I try to stick with companies whose products I've tried and experienced good results with.

Another reason people don't get the results they desire is the advertising hype surrounding supplements. Let me let you in on a little secret: many of the industry ads are lies. More often than not, the well-chiseled guys and bikini-clad, body-fat-free women whose photos grace the labels on supplement bottles never even used these products to attain their current physiques. Some have even used a health-risking chemical cocktail of illegal anabolic steroids stacked with fat-burning drugs.

I'm assuming that, like myself, you'd rather build your own ultimate body in a natural, healthy way, so don't get taken in by these ads. While I don't believe it's an unrealistic goal to look like some of the models on the packaging, often taking the advertised product isn't the way to get there. On a personal note, it just makes me so angry to see the frustration many of these products cause when someone new to fitness wastes money buying into the hype of these ads and then quits his or her training program when he or she doesn't end up looking like the models.

## JOHN-ISM

FMS's goal is to make you better, not turn you into someone else or have you conform to a media-hyped ideal, but to help you be the best you can be.

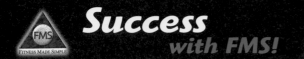
I am a 35-year-old accountant. I began your *Six Pack Abs* routine about four weeks ago with the intention of getting back in shape and I am seeing results fast!

Your program has all the elements I was looking for in an ab routine: it is simple, moves quickly, and gives instant results. The nutritional tips are also very helpful.

I had been in good shape at one point in my life; I played four years of soccer in college. My life progressed to marriage, a daughter, and a great job behind a desk! The only problem with a desk job is that it is easy to get out of shape. My coworkers are following my progress and have seen my before-and-after pictures. Several of them have become inspired to get back in shape as well. I've encouraged them to use the FMS plan.

Hopefully, my testimony will be an inspiration to someone else. Thank you for sharing your knowledge.

## MY THREE RULES FOR TAKING SUPPLEMENTS

How can you make sure supplements improve your body and not just the supplement companies' bottom lines? Here are three simple rules I follow.

### 1. Don't Use More than Two Supplements at a Time

Don't go crazy, the way some people do, by taking too many supplements at once. If you do, you'll never know which product is doing what. If I'm going to use supplements, I may try one fat-burning product and one muscle-building product for a few weeks at a time to see what results, if any, they're capable of bringing me.

## 2. Stick with Supplements That Give You "Cosmetically Significant" Results

Very few supplements produce what I call *cosmetically significant* results. These are results you can actually see and feel. A lot of times you'll see ads that say, "Our products produce 100 percent more fat loss than a placebo." They're not necessarily lying—they could in fact have an appreciably accurate scientific study. If you look closely at that study, however, you may find out that the control group lost an average of one pound while the group taking the supplement lost an average of two pounds. That is a 100 percent increase—however, *ain't nobody gonna notice a two-pound loss on a 200-pound guy; ain't nobody gonna notice that on a 120-pound woman, either.*

That's why I only care about cosmetically significant results. Don't worry about the numbers. Don't get caught up in the hype. Just pay attention to what the product you're taking is doing for you.

## 3. If You Don't See Results in a Couple of Weeks, Try Something Else

With any supplement you try, if you don't notice some sort of change within a two-week time period, in my opinion you're wasting your money. Manufacturers say, "Oh, but you have to take our products for three months to see results." Of course they say that, because they want you to shell out money for three months. Trust me: if you've been taking a supplement for two months and 29 days with no results, you're not going to magically see a revolutionary change when you wake up the next morning to reach the end of that third month. Try a product for a couple of weeks. If you don't get at least a hint of the results you want, move on to something else.

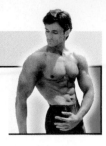

## JOHN-ISM

It doesn't matter where you start out. What matters is where you end up and that you enjoy the journey.

# MY FAVORITE SUPPLEMENTS

The following are a few supplements that in some way have helped me and thousands of other Fitness Made Simple customers achieve our fat-burning and lean-muscle-building goals.

One further note about the supplement business: it changes faster than the electronics industry or fashion world, with old products disappearing daily and new ones constantly being introduced. That's why, instead of brand names, I've listed here the active ingredients that I look for in a supplement—the things that have proven themselves worthy to me over the years.

There are a total of eight different supplements. The first three are for fat burning, the next two are primarily used for increasing muscle mass, and the last three are what I like to call *general health-enhancing supplements* that can also benefit your overall fitness lifestyle. Each of these supplements works better for some people than others, so you may have to experiment to find which products work best for you.

### Fat-Burning Supplements

**PYRUVATE.** One fat-burning supplement I like is called pyruvate, which is a naturally occurring end product of our bodies' metabolism of sugar and starch. It helps to increase energy *and* stimulate fat loss. Pyruvate is believed to work its magic by prioritizing the transport of nutrients after meals to muscle cells rather than to fat cells, thereby increasing glycogen, otherwise known as "muscle fuel," reserves for energy while decreasing fat deposition.

It may further enhance fat loss by increasing metabolism and thermogenesis as well as by improving insulin sensitivity. Pyruvate is one of the hottest fat-burning products on the market now, but *not all forms are created equal.* Since quality pyruvate is very hard to find and many bogus brands come out with impure, low-grade forms of the product, I always stick with brands that have proven their effectiveness to me in the past. Pyruvate works well to keep me lean, and it's a very good alternative for people who can't tolerate the stimulatory properties of other fat-burning products.

**GUGGULSTERONES.** This is another stimulant-free, fat-burning supplement. I know, it sounds more like a medical condition you'd rather avoid than a fat-loss supplement. It's actually a unique ingredient designed to optimize the function of our metabolisms as well as support low cholesterol levels. High-potency guggulsterones help stimulate the thyroid gland to produce more thyroid hormones. This action not only results in a healthier, more active thyroid but also works to keep our basal metabolic rates (BMRs) at a higher level, even when we're following a lower-caloric meal plan. This is a time when thyroid activity and metabolism can decrease, causing fat loss to slow down or seemingly stop completely. With a high BMR more calories are burned and more weight is lost. Sounds pretty simple.

Guggulsterones also have a few added benefits. As metabolic regulators, they help improve skin conditions, like acne, by decreasing the number and size of blemishes, and they provide the skin with specific nutrients that promote a clear, soft, and healthy appearance. Guggulsterones also help support lowered LDL, or "bad," cholesterol and triglyceride levels while maintaining high levels of HDL, or "good," cholesterol. For a synergistic fat-loss effect and to maximize results, it's often recommended to stack guggulsterones with other fat burners like pyruvate.

The best thing I like about guggulsterones is that they help me get over that plateau, or sticking point, where I stop losing fat even if I drop my calories lower and lower. The metabolic boost is very helpful at that time.

**EVODIAMINE.** According to studies, evodiamine—an extract from the plant *Evodia rutaecarpa*, which is found in Chinese provinces—has been shown to elevate body heat production and increase resting core temperature so more fat can be burned at rest. It may also inhibit the growth and metastases of certain cancer cells in vitro and influence the secretion of catecholamines from the adrenal glands.

I've found evodiamine to be one of the most effective fat-loss ingredients I've ever used, which is one reason I had it included, along with several other metabolism-boosting ingredients, in the FMS PAC (Power Ab Chiseler) ATTACK, a supplement product many FMS followers have used. FMS PAC ATTACK also contains green tea leaf extract, 5-HTP, ginseng extract, and yohimbine, all of which have been shown to boost metabolism, increase calorie burning, or reduce appetite. This sort of biogenic amine blend promotes thermogenesis for maximum fat burning. I find FMS PAC ATTACK to be the best fat-fighting supplement on the market today.

## Muscle-Building Supplements

**GLUTAMINE.** If I had to limit myself to only one muscle-building supplement, this would be it. I personally find glutamine to be the single-best overall product for people involved in sports and weight training. Its benefits even extend into the fat-burning and general health-enhancing categories as well.

Glutamine has been around in vitamin stores forever and is probably the most underrated physique-enhancement supplement on the market today. Glutamine is an amino acid, which does many good things. It has been shown to decrease catabolism (muscle breakdown), increase growth hormone levels, reduce body-fat deposition, and lead to better muscle recovery, growth, and protein synthesis. In fact it's called the "anti-overtraining" supplement since it's very effective at preserving muscle mass when people are following a lower-calorie, fat-burning nutrition plan like the one I laid out earlier.

When I'm using it, I take one to two teaspoons of glutamine daily, and I like to cycle it six weeks on and four weeks off (that means I take it for six weeks then stop for four weeks). I've noticed that if I continually use any supplement without cycling off it for a while, my body adjusts to it. My results diminish while my cash outlay for the product remains the same. Giving my body a bit of a rest allows it to normalize before reintroducing a supplement back into my program. I take one teaspoon of glutamine blended in a protein shake with my post-workout meal to replenish glycogen reserves and, I hope, increase protein synthesis during this important muscle-mass recovery and growth period. I sometimes take an additional teaspoon mixed in water about an hour prior to workouts for strength increases and better pumps.

**CREATINE.** Creatine is one of the most popular muscle-building supplements on the market and with good reason. It's great for hydrating the muscles, which increases bulk, strength, and energy. Creatine occurs naturally in our skeletal systems and helps supply energy to muscle cells. We also get creatine from food, mostly meat and fish. In recent years creatine supplementation has been used not only by people looking to build muscle but also as a therapy for certain neurological and neuromuscular diseases.

In my experience creatine is best when you're in a building phase; I've found it's less effective when I'm trying to cut up. That's because, at least with me, in addition to hydrating the muscles, creatine also causes my body to hold some water between the skin and muscle layers, which creates a puffy, smooth look. That's something no one wants when trying to maximize definition. I also don't find it's necessary to do a loading phase with creatine, as some suggest. I simply take one serving per day after my workout for best results.

## General Health-Enhancing Supplements

While the list of available fitness, bodybuilding, and fat-loss supplements can go on and on, the list of those that have proven beneficial to me doesn't. There are just three other products that I use regularly and that I actually think of as staples in my nutrition plan.

**WHEY PROTEIN.** I don't look at this as a supplement at all; instead, it's just another protein food option similar to chicken breasts, water-packed tuna, and egg whites. Whey protein is great because it's a quick, convenient, and tasty way to increase my protein intake without having to cook. It's versatile and easily combined with frozen fruits or fat-free, sugar-free pudding mixes to make a seemingly endless variety of shakes. Some of my friends even use it to make high-protein muffins and cakes. Also, nitrogen retention from the hydrolyzed whey peptides contained in these powders has been shown to be 16 times greater than that of free-form amino acids and nearly twice that of whole foods. When I need protein to be absorbed fast, like after workouts, whey protein is a great quick fix.

I do want to point out that when I say "protein powders" I'm talking about the ones that are around 80 to 100 or so calories per serving and contain primarily protein and a gram or so of carbs and fat. I'm *not* talking about those weight-gain powders that are advertised all over and contain 2,000-plus calories per serving. I tried some of these when I was first starting out, and I think they should change the name of that category of supplements to fat-gain powders because that's all they ever did for me. Yeah, they added pounds—to my waistline and that's it. Most are primarily carbs, and as far as I'm concerned, you may as well take up residence at the local bakery and eat the caloric equivalent in brownies. At least it would be a tastier way to gain weight.

Some Fitness Made Simple members who are following a high-protein, definition-enhancing meal plan even use whey protein shakes as a meal replacement in between their solid food meals.

**FLAX MEAL.** To me flax meal is similar to whey protein. I consider it more of a food option than a supplement, and the benefits are numerous. For starters flax meal is one of the best sources anywhere of fatty acids, including alpha linolenic acid, omega-3 essential fatty acids, and omega-6 essential fatty acids. All are extremely beneficial for your heart. In particular omega-3s have been shown to decrease risk of arrhythmias, which can lead to sudden cardiac death; decrease triglyceride levels; decrease the growth rate of atherosclerotic plaque; and even lower blood pressure slightly. Omega-3s may also help with arthritis, reduce skin problems such as acne, and temper the effects of stress.

Additionally, flax meal is a great source of fiber, which is crucial to your digestive system. One challenge of following a high-protein meal plan, as I call for in the Fitness Made Simple nutrition program, is potential constipation. This not only feels uncomfortable but can also cause a protrusion in your abdominal area. By getting a high level of fiber in your diet, however, you can avoid constipation and keep your digestive system healthy. I believe a well-functioning digestive system is a key factor in building a lean, muscular body.

Finally, as we discussed in earlier chapters, the fats in flax meal slow down the absorption of high GI foods, thus decreasing fat-producing insulin spikes. I like to sprinkle some flax meal into protein shakes, oatmeal, and low-fat yogurt.

## JOHN-ISM

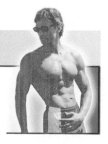

Consistency is key to achieving results. You can't just eat right or work out one day.

Dear FMS,

I'm writing this letter to say thanks for sharing your knowledge of how to take care of our bodies even with little free time for ourselves.

I have two jobs and I work seven days a week. I used to go to the gym once in a while, but this frequency was decreasing more and more, and I ended up paying the gym for months without even going.

I kept seeing the Fitness Made Simple commercials over and over again, and I finally made up my mind to try it. I started the workout and what I love about it is that John makes it easy for you. At first I thought, *That's it?* But then the next morning my abs were burning like crazy. It was such a *great* feeling! After I realized this, I exercised every day and adopted the recommended diet that John talks about.

I was astonished to see the results in the mirror after just three months! My waist went from 35 inches to 30 inches and my weight from 175 pounds to 152 pounds. I literally had to buy a new pair of jeans because my old ones were too big. I lost more than 10 percent of body fat, and not only did my abs start to show, but I noticed that my whole body changed. I became leaner and looked better than ever!

So thank you, Fitness Made Simple. You have definitely changed my life! I highly support Fitness Made Simple and highly recommend it to anyone at any age if you want to be in the best shape of your life.

**MULTIVITAMIN PLUS.** By "plus," I mean a multivitamin that gives you more than the RDA of most vitamins. Active people following a fitness lifestyle have different needs than most couch potatoes. Regular exercise can create more free radicals and place more stress on your body. The right multivitamin formulation, one with antioxidants and metabolism boosters, can help you protect yourself against that. In a perfect world, of course, we'd get all the vitamins and minerals we need through food. Thanks to soil depletion and other factors, however, not all foods today contain the essential ingredients we think they do. Taking a multivitamin plus is like added insurance that you're getting all the vitamins and minerals your body requires. That's why I helped to develop the FMS Power Multi-Vitamin, which incorporates all of these benefits.

# CHANGE YOUR BODY, CHANGE YOUR LIFE

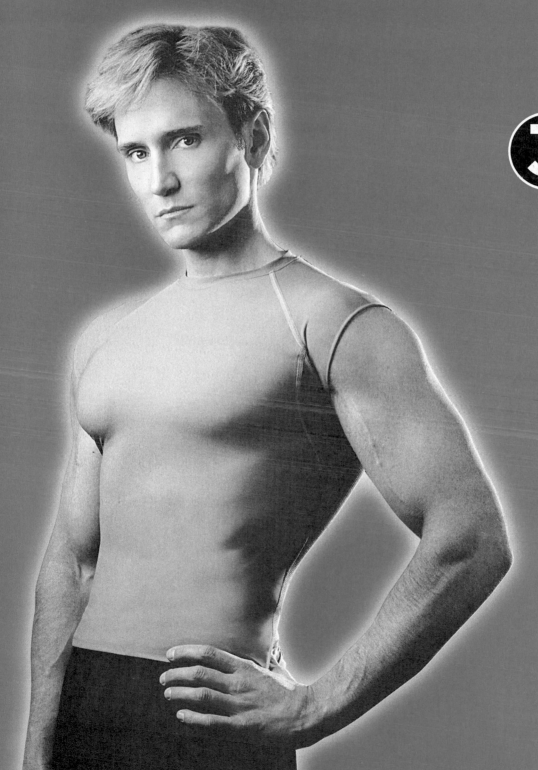

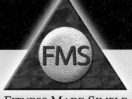

FITNESS MADE SIMPLE

# FITNESS MADE
# PERMANENT

We've reached what may be the most important chapter in this entire book, covering how to take everything you've learned and put it into action *permanently*. I've shown you how to change your body for the better; now I want to show you how to change your life forever.

Over the years I've received dozens of letters from people asking for help in sticking with an exercise or diet plan, but one from a lady named Ronnie, who'd just ordered a Fitness Made Simple video, really hit me. To make a long story short, Ronnie had recently started watching what she was eating and had plans to join a neighborhood gym.

Unfortunately, Thanksgiving and multiple holiday parties came along, and with them came an unwanted eight pounds. Ronnie found herself drowning in feelings of frustration and failure, the same emotions she experienced on previous efforts to stick with diet and exercise plans. She was reaching out for help to make the new year different.

I could relate to Ronnie's frustration, and I bet you can, too. In my experience up to 90 percent of people who resolve to do something end up not achieving their goals, especially fitness-related ones. Why? Because they give up on them. The fitness industry counts on this. I think if every well-intentioned person who signed up for a gym membership actually went on a regular basis, that gym would probably exceed occupancy regulations, or, at the very least, there'd be an interminable wait to get on the stair-climber.

So now that you know what to do to get your body in shape, how do you make sure you do it? Now that you have the key to a better body, how do you make sure the door stays open? I'll share with you what I shared with Ronnie—the rules that worked for me.

# MY SIX RULES FOR STICKING WITH A FITNESS PLAN

When it comes to long-term success, these six rules proved invaluable to me.

### 1. Make Fitness a Priority and Readjust Your Mind-Set

Everyone complains about time limitations. People justify not working out or eating healthy by saying, "I don't have time." If this is the case, you have to *make* time.

It's not that hard to do. Think of fitness as a priority, something that you must fit in, like going to work, eating, sleeping, or even using the bathroom.

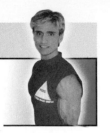

## JOHN-ISM

Don't ever accept "no" as a *final* answer to anything you want, and never take "no" as an answer from someone who doesn't have the authority to say "yes."

It should be that much of a staple. Everyone has 24 hours in a day. That's a lot of time. What matters is how you fill those hours. Take a moment to list all of the things you're doing now that you make time for and ask yourself how important they are to you and your happiness. Are they more important than improving your health and getting the body you want? More important than feeling better? When I used this simple technique, I couldn't believe how many ridiculous, habitual things I was unknowingly filling my days with and putting ahead of my fitness pursuits.

To further solidify your commitment to improving your body, take a page out of Oprah's book. She wrote a contract with herself. I didn't go that far. I just wrote down my short-term and long-term goals as well as what I planned to do to accomplish them. Writing things down just makes them seem more real.

## 2. Make It Real: Give Yourself Something Tangible to Focus On

The fact that you're holding this book in your hands is a great start, both mentally and physically, to making fitness a permanent part of your life. Mentally, it's something you can see, feel, and touch, and it represents your commitment to putting ideas into practice. Most of us have amazing thoughts every day, but only a select few ever act on them. You'll notice those few are usually the most successful.

## JOHN-ISM

Fitness is an investment you make in yourself, and it's one that pays off with a lifetime of benefits.

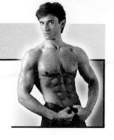

Physically, Fitness Made Simple provides the exact time-conserving workout routine and nutritional meal plan thousands of women and men, including myself, have used to attain their fat-burning and lean muscle-building goals. I've been told it's like having a personal trainer on hand 24 hours a day providing you with the complete blueprint for creating a toned, defined physique. In just eight weeks this program helped me develop the tight six-pack of abs I'd always wanted but never was able to see before, despite years of trying.

This book isn't the only way to make your goals tangible, of course. Joining a gym or buying inexpensive home exercise equipment like free weights and a bench are two more ways you can show commitment to your goal.

### 3. Take Photos

No matter how out of shape you think you are, take a "before" photo prior to beginning your workout regimen and additional snapshots every two weeks until you reach your goal. This practice can be nerve-racking, but nothing beats it when it comes to keeping your mind on your goal. It provides a starting point and biweekly reminders of your progress. I find it difficult to notice improvements on a day-to-day basis, which wreaks havoc on my motivation. When I compare periodic photos and notice the benefits of my efforts, however, I feel much more satisfied and strengthen my resolve.

### 4. Practice Nutritional Planning

"Good eating" takes no more time than "bad eating," but it does require a small—and I emphasize *small*—amount of planning. This is why I suggest taking a few minutes one day and writing down all the foods you want to keep in your nutrition plan and then shopping for them one day each week. I also think it's helpful to cook one day a week and refrigerate or freeze some meals for later in the week. For instance, since I love bulk discount stores like Costco and Sam's Club, I get the jumbo chicken breast packages and cook two of them on Sundays, storing serving-size portions of the tasty morsels in my refrigerator for use throughout the week. When needed I take them out, add some brown rice or a sweet potato (previously cooked) and/or vegetables, pack this nutritious meal in a plastic container, and carry it with me to eat later in the day. This practice benefits both my muscle definition and my wallet when compared to the often pricey, sugar-laden, and saturated-fat-filled fast-food fixes I might have succumbed to.

Speaking of fast food, nowadays it can be a help rather than a hindrance in keeping our physiques lean and muscular. Just select healthy alternatives. As stated earlier, most major franchises offer low-fat fare, and it doesn't take any more time to select the chicken breast salad combo over the bacon double cheeseburger or to opt for the chicken soft taco with sauce on the side instead of the deep-fried cheese tortilla. You can also carry convenient protein powders, meal replacements, and nutrition bars with you so you don't fall victim to fast-food cravings. If you just think about what you're putting into your mouth, eating on the go doesn't have to translate into eating badly.

Planning what you want to eat and making smart choices when you're eating out gives you control—and control will help you get the body you've been dreaming of.

## 5. Make Good Eating the Rule and Cheating the Exception

I said it before and it bears repeating: as long as you eat "clean" by following your FMS nutrition plan the majority of the time, the truth is that one day of indulgence in most cases will have no lasting visible impact on the gains you've made over several weeks of good days.

Dear John,

I would like to share the way Fitness Made Simple has truly changed the way I look and feel. I went from a size 8 to a size 4–6. I am 5'7", and I have lost 9 pounds thus far (151 pounds to 142 pounds). Before FMS, I would exercise a few times a week, but I was not looking the way I wished. I wanted to become tighter and leaner, but I was not accomplishing those goals. Now I can see more definition in my legs, arms, back, chest, shoulders, and butt. The way my clothes fit has changed dramatically, and I'm well on my way to the body I've always wanted.

Strength training at a heart-pumping cardio pace is the key to my new physique. In addition to changing the way I look, the program has

## 6. Don't Be Too Hard on Yourself

No one eats perfectly all the time, so don't give up if you have a bad meal, a bad day, even a bad week. The same is true with exercise. There are going to be days when you may not feel like doing your A.M. cardio workout or lifting weights later. If that happens and you miss a day, don't give up and tell yourself it's hopeless. Just try to make progress the next day.

Once again, keep in mind that the first few weeks of anything new can be difficult. You're trying to change a lifetime of habits, and it can't be done in a single day. It's crucial to look at your new fitness lifestyle as just that—a lifestyle. Trust that you are taking control of your life and changing it for the better. Look to the future with a sense of eagerness and excitement!

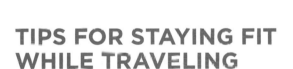

changed the way I feel. I am more confident,
I have more energy, and I seek out new challenges
and inspiration. I think of your words often:
"train hard, eat right, rest well, and you can
attain all your fitness goals." How true this is!!
It is awe inspiring that something so simple
can have such far-reaching effects.

You are truly an inspiration for me.
Thanks for sharing and stay well!

# TIPS FOR STAYING FIT
# WHILE TRAVELING

Quite often I've found my butt on an airplane, something I look forward to
with the same enthusiasm as a dental appointment, traveling to and from
various personal appearances. Since I do spokesmodel work for different
companies, they fly me around to fitness, bodybuilding, and nutrition expo-
sitions to sign photos, answer workout/meal plan questions, and basically
represent them to industry members and the general public. Usually these
conventions are spaced apart throughout the year so they're a nice break
in my routine. Sometimes, though, they come in a schedule-shattering,
cross-country cluster from Atlanta to Los Angeles. How do you stay in shape

during such a hectic travel schedule? I'm sure this thought has entered the minds of more than a few of you frequent flyers out there. It might also have passed right through them once you realized solving the dilemma requires a little bit of thought and planning. Fortunately, I can share my personal experiences in the form of a few tips to help you stay fit while on the go.

## 1. Prepare a Carry-On Meal for Your Travel Day

If you're looking for lots of sodium, sugar, and saturated fat, airline food might be the way to go. I think the buttery sauce on the "sautéed chicken nasty" they almost served me one time could actually have equaled my daily allotment of fat grams. Add to that the salted peanuts coupled with the high glycemic piece of cake, and I'd be nicely bloated by landing time. Thanks to a little preplanning, however, I now bring plastic containers with a grilled chicken breast and mixed vegetables to keep me from resorting to airline cuisine. On one flight I even heard an envious passenger a couple of rows behind me breathe a sigh of regret as he said to his seatmate, "That looks a heck of a lot better than what we got." If you're not into cooking, as I'm usually not, you can also simply pick up a healthful meal, like a chicken or turkey breast salad on pita, to go from the drive-through window of many popular fast-food restaurants. You'll notice just about all the major franchises are now catering to fitness folk with special high-protein, low-fat food options.

Bringing my own food on the plane has two benefits. First, it helps me stick to my nutrition plan. Second, it helps me mentally stay in control of the situation and keeps me focused right from the start that this trip doesn't have to interfere with my fitness program.

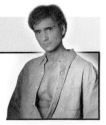

## JOHN-ISM

Don't let other people impose their limitations on your abilities.

## 2. Make Sure Your Hotel Has a Gym

This one is very important. The first thing I do when I get my itinerary is to call the hotel to make sure it has some sort of workout facility. It doesn't have to be fancy. Just a lifecycle, elliptical trainer, or treadmill for my morning cardio and a multistation universal gym for some basic weight training suits me fine for short trips. I get to stay in the exercise mode while getting a break from my normal routine. Surprisingly, I sometimes return home in better shape, tighter and more defined, than when I left. Because I have a tendency to overtrain a bit, I guess this abbreviated travel routine gives my body a needed rest and my muscles a chance to fill out.

If your hotel doesn't have a gym, like some of the no-frills ones I've been put in, you still have a couple of other training options. Number 1, check out local gyms, some of which usually have deals open to fitness-oriented hotel guests. Ask someone at the front desk for details. Number 2, use your room. Remember, exercises using your own body weight, like push-ups and stomach crunches, can help you stay pumped and get blood flowing to those working muscles. Of course, for cardiovascular activity there's always walking and jogging. These are also great ways to see the area where you're staying, a feat that's otherwise difficult for me considering I'm stuck inside convention halls most of the day.

I'd also like to recommend that no matter what exercise you're planning, make it a priority. Try to do a good portion of it first thing in the morning to ensure you get it in. Too many times the days tend to get away from us when we're traveling, and if we put off working out until the later hours, it often gets left out completely.

## 3. Eating Healthy While Traveling Is No More Difficult than Eating Poorly

If even the fast-food places offer low-fat, low-calorie food options, there's no excuse for straying from your nutrition plan while you're away. As I always say, eating well takes no more time than eating badly. It just requires that

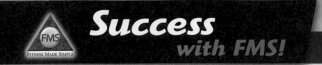
Dear FMS,

I'd like to tell you how the Fitness Made Simple program contributed to a significant change in my physique. My desire to lose weight and get in shape became most critical when, at age 13, I hit a peak of 215 pounds on my 5'9" frame. I was at the end of eighth grade, preparing to enter high school that fall, and I wanted to play on the football team. With football camp a few months away, I knew I would never get through it if I didn't begin to get into shape.

With the help of my parents I began a healthy diet, and we joined a fitness club for exercise. I then saw John Basedow's infomercial and how great he looks and I decided to start Fitness Made Simple. I was able to incorporate FMS into my fitness regimen, and, as an added advantage, it was beneficial for my off-season football training as well. I am extremely happy with the results of John's program. *When I look in the mirror, I still can't believe it's me.* With the help of FMS, I was able to bring my physique

you take a moment to think about what you're putting in your mouth. Stay in control by practicing some discipline, and you'll thank yourself for it when you get home.

## 4. Don't Forget Your Supplements

We've already established that traveling doesn't have to translate into a vacation or deviation from our fitness lifestyles. So if you're currently using any supplements, there's no reason not to bring them with you.

to a higher level of definition, and I have made the FMS exercises part of my regular workouts.

It is now two years since I started my fitness program, and I weigh *145 pounds!* As you can see from my photos, I am in the best shape I could be. My life has changed so much. I am full of energy and confident about how I look. *When I look back, I realize how getting in shape was very difficult in the beginning but, with the help of people like John demonstrating that it can be done, I was inspired to keep trying.* With this in mind, I am hoping that my story can inspire other teens to use the Fitness Made Simple programs to lose weight and get into shape. With the number of overweight teens hitting an alarming rate, hopefully my story could be a wake-up call and put others on the road to fitness and good health.

My deepest thanks to John and Fitness Made Simple!!

Following as much of your usual daily schedule as possible will help keep you in the fitness mode while traveling so that by the time you return home, you might just be in even better shape than when you left.

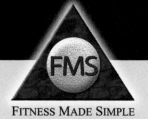

FITNESS MADE SIMPLE

# THE POWER TO BE BETTER

Today's failure has no bearing on tomorrow's success.

You may remember that John-ism—it was how I started this book and it's how I want to end it. In my mind no phrase is more powerful. It tells us that no matter what's happened in the past or how low we feel in the present, nothing is ever impossible in the future. Once you take control of your body, you start taking control of your life, and then anything you can dream you can do.

When I think back to that miserable Christmas years ago, when I started to turn my own life around, it sometimes seems like only yesterday, but in other ways it feels like a lifetime ago. That's true not only when I see how I look but also when I think about how I now spend my days. As I often say, fitness has a ripple effect on our lives, and there's no better proof of that than me.

My old life—one filled with frustration, anxiety, and avoiding other people—is dead and buried. It's on the trash heap right next to the wrappers from all those burgers and brownies I used to devour. In its place I have an exciting new life—one occupied by shooting videos, creating TV shows, writing books, and making personal appearances. It's hard work, but I'm living my dream. More important, I'm helping other men and women realize *their* dreams. Everywhere I go, people come up to me and thank me for helping them. They tell me amazing stories about how Fitness Made Simple transformed their bodies and lives, making them more energetic, more confident, and happier. You've seen some of their stories in these pages as well. I'm flattered that people recognize me, but even more thrilling is seeing the impact that a few small positive changes can have on someone's life.

What are your dreams? I know that if you stick with Fitness Made Simple, it will help you make miraculous changes in your life. Some of those will be physical changes—your love handles or flabby thighs will disappear, you'll get the muscle definition you've been longing for, you'll cut your risk for disease, and you'll feel better. Even more amazing, though, are the changes that will take place in the rest of your life. Once you get your body in shape, I believe—no, I *know*—that you'll stop settling in every single part of your life, from your job to your relationships. You'll have escaped from the land of "good enough." You'll have discovered the cure for settle-itis, and you'll know that it doesn't come from a bottle or even a book. It comes from inside you.

I want to end with Bryan's story. Bryan was about to get married, and he promised his fiancée that he would be in shape by their wedding day. Given the way his body looked at the time, that was going to be no easy feat. Still,

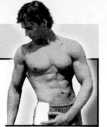

## JOHN-ISM

You will never rise above the image you have of yourself; perception is everything. Reality is what you make it. Don't focus on the way you are—focus on the way you want to be.

Bryan started the Fitness Made Simple program and, just like I suggest, took a new photo of himself every single week. He saw results pretty quickly, and as each week went by, he found himself getting more and more motivated, which just kept improving his results. Flipping through the pictures of Bryan, it was like seeing a new person every week.

Finally, his wedding day arrived and Bryan had achieved his goal: the body of his dreams. He was ecstatic, of course, not only about the way he looked but also that he had kept his promise to his new wife. As he told me, "It changed my life, John. It's hard to put all that into words, but it really has changed my life."

Just like it will change yours.

Dear FMS,

My name is Bryan and I am a 35-year-old father of two.

I had been working out since I was about 25, but somewhere around three to four years ago, I must have started to let myself go. It was such a gradual thing I didn't notice it happening; however, I realized how much I'd changed this past January. You see, I was getting married in July, and my fiancée, Carey, and her bridesmaids were looking for a wedding dress. The girls all got together one day to help Carey pick out a dress or at least get an idea from magazines. They started passing around a magazine with a ripped guy in it and going nuts over how hot he was. I turned to Carey and said, "I look like that, don't I, honey?" to which she replied, giggling, "You mean you used to." That's when I realized all the "extra me" I was carrying around. So in front of my fiancée and all the bridesmaids, I stated that by the wedding I would look like that guy in the magazine. The next day I woke up and thought, *how am I gonna pull this off?* I watched one of John's commercials on TV that morning and decided I wanted to be one of his FMS Success Stories, too.

That's when I modified my diet, started John's workouts, and took a picture to mark my starting point, just as John suggests. As two weeks passed I started to wonder if I was really losing anything. This is where the pictures come in. I reluctantly asked Carey to take my two-week picture, not expecting to see a difference, but when I compared the first

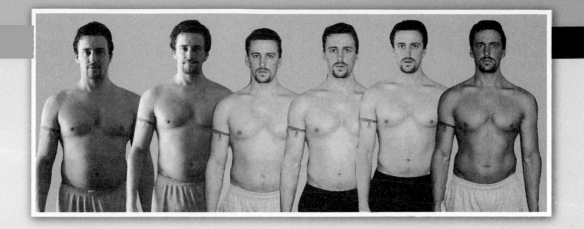

picture to the new one, wow, what a difference! I could see the changes starting already. This gave me renewed inspiration, and the same kind of thing happened every two weeks. That's what showed me how much Fitness Made Simple really works. The next thing that really surprised me was how much energy I had. I didn't feel like sleeping all day.

The way John approaches everything makes it fun and it never seems like a chore to work out. I actually look forward to that part of my day. By the wedding day I had kept my promise thanks to John and FMS, and I had a renewed feeling of self-esteem. On our honeymoon I was able to walk around the beaches with my shirt off and feel good about it! When I started the FMS programs I was 208 pounds with a waist measurement of 38 inches. After just 11 weeks I weighed 183 pounds and my waist had dropped down to 34.5 inches. Now, 18 weeks from the date I started following John's simple tips, I am down to 178 pounds. That's 30 pounds I shed off. Wow! As an added bonus I have lots more muscle tone, too.

I know it is only going to get better from here. Thanks, John!!!

# INDEX

Entries in *italics* refer to recipes.

# ABOUT THE AUTHOR

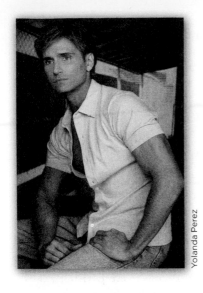

Yolanda Perez

Well, if you own a TV, you're probably aware of fitness celebrity John Basedow and his ubiquitous commercials for the bestselling Fitness Made Simple video series, which has helped improve the bodies and lives of thousands of men and women. From starting out in his parents' basement to being seen on television sets across the country to being deemed a "pop culture icon" by the media, John's journey is an American dream come true, rags-to-riches story.

Fueled by an undying persistence and his personal motto "believe in yourself and you can accomplish anything," John has achieved international recognition and created a media empire with Fitness Made Simple, which includes DVDs, CDs, supplements, commercials, and infomercials, all aimed at raising awareness about the importance of making fitness a part of your life. He's been featured on numerous TV and radio shows as well as in print media ranging from the *Los Angeles Times* to the *National Examiner*. In fact, the *New York Times* places him alongside NASCAR and figure skating in the contemporary pantheon of "great American sports television phenomena," and *Muscle & Fitness* magazine named him the top infomercial star of the past 20 years.

In addition to being a model who's graced the pages of just about every major exercise magazine, John's also a widely respected columnist who's written articles for more than a dozen publications. He's a frequently requested fitness expert who appears each month on dozens of radio programs across the country, and he hosts "Work It Out Wednesdays with John Basedow" on WMJC-FM 94.3 in New York.

Recently, a television production company offered John his own unique reality series, "John Basedow TV," which is based on John's life. Building on his nationwide popularity, "John Basedow TV" is a feel-good show that delivers John's positive message for your body and mind in a creative, engaging way with a rare mix of inspirational and comedic elements.

Even with such a full schedule, John makes time to help out various charities, including the American Heart Association and American Diabetes Association, as well as to motivate others to follow their dreams with his popular "Power to Change Your Body and Life" seminars. As John says, "If you can think it, you can do it. Don't listen to negative people. If you listen only to your inner self, work hard, and never quit, you can achieve anything."

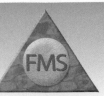
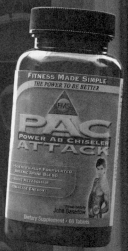